Thai Massage

Richard Gold PhD LAc

In 1972, Richard Gold graduated from Oberlin College with a BA degree in World Religions. He graduated from New England School of Acupuncture in 1978. Since then, he has devoted himself to studying, practicing and teaching oriental medicine. He holds a Doctorate in Psychology. Richard has participated in advanced studies in acupuncture in Shanghai, China, in 1980 and in Shiatsu in Osaka, Japan, in 1986. His studies in traditional Thai medical massage began in 1988 in Chiang Mai, Thailand. Richard is a founding Board member of the International Professional School of Bodywork and the Pacific College of Oriental Medicine in San Diego, California, and also of the Pacific Institute of Oriental Medicine in New York City. He divides his time between private practice, teaching, writing, family and gardening in San Diego, California.

For Churchill Livingstone:

Commissioning editor: Inta Ozols
Project manager: Valerie Burgess
Project editor: Valerie Dearing
Project controller: Derek Robertson
Design: Judith Wright
Copy editor: Stephanie Pickering
Promotions manager: Hilary Brown

Thai Massage

A TRADITIONAL MEDICAL TECHNIQUE

Richard Gold PhD LAc
Practitioner and Lecturer, San Diego, California, USA

Foreword by

Ted J. Kaptchuk OMD
Instructor in Medicine, Harvard Medical School
Associate Director, Centre for Alternative Medical Research,
Beth Israel Deaconess Medical Center, Boston,
Massachusetts, USA

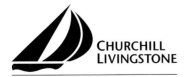

CHURCHILL
LIVINGSTONE

EDINBURGH LONDON NEW YORK PHILADELPHIA SAN FRANCISCO SYDNEY TORONTO 1998

CHURCHILL LIVINGSTONE
A Division of Harcourt Brace and Company Limited

Churchill Livingstone, Robert Stevenson House, 1–3 Baxter's Place, Leith Walk, Edinburgh EH1 3AF, UK

First published 1998

ISBN 0 443 05935 7

British Library Cataloguing in Publication Data
A catalogue record for this book is available from the British Library.

Library of Congress Cataloging in Publication Data
A catalog record for this book is available from the Library of Congress

Produced by Longman Singapore Publishers (Pte) Ltd.,
Printed in Singapore

Contents

Foreword

Dr Richard Gold's new volume on traditional Thai massage comes at an auspicious moment in the history of health care. For a long time, the words 'cosmopolitan medicine' have meant the biological science-based medicine that developed primarily in Western Europe and North America.[1] Until recently, this biomedical approach to illness and health has been the only common denominator for health care available in most urban centers throughout the world. All other medical systems or practices were regional or indigenous.

In the last 20 years, the ethnocentricity of the world has diminished and (excluding fundamentalist and racist trends) there exists a new openness to the experiences, knowledge and wisdom of multiple cultures. This is especially true of health care. Acupuncture and other forms of East Asian medicine are now available in every major city on every continent.[2,3] Ayurvedic medicine has ceased to be confined to the Indian subcontinent and is almost as easily available as Oriental medicine.[2] Alternative and unconventional western versions of health care have also spread across the globe. Homeopathy is now widely available throughout the world.[4,5] Chiropractic, the most indigenous American healing art, has established itself as an integral part of health care systems in major centers on every continent.[6,7] Cosmopolitan medicine has ceased to be the product of one epistemology and has become a concept in flux.

This volume is especially important because of this global shift. At what point does a local tradition become integrated into the broadly available medicine of the entire planet? How is this managed? In what way is this valuable? Who decides? The traditional medicine of Thailand is an important test case. Outside of Thai culture, for a long time, it has been mostly an intellectual and academic secret (for example, see references 8 and 9). Few major presentations have been undertaken to make Thai medicine accessible to the general public and/or professional health care providers.

Dr Gold's new book is a critical step towards filling this void. He has presented the traditional approach to hands-on healing and bodywork that has long been essential to the traditional medicine of Thailand. For the first time, this dimension of Thai health care has an opportunity to make its voice heard in the world arena. What we encounter in this volume is a thoughtful, coherent, respectful and profound method of healing. Dr Gold's book presents the reader and professional health care provider with both a challenge and an opportunity. How we respond to Dr Gold's transmission will help formulate the vital question of how a new cosmopolitan tradition will be formulated in the 21st century.

Dr Gold's book comes at an auspicious moment for another reason. Health care is rediscovering the value of touch, bodywork and massage. Advanced technology, sophisticated pharmacology, and even 'holistic' approaches with herbs, acupuncture or psychotherapy, still omit a vital component of what many people need for healing. Medical historians have speculated that massage may be the oldest form of healing.[10] Massage is now undergoing a renaissance and re-emerging as a critical component of medicine. The archaic depths of the implications of being touched to promote healing and maintain health are asserting themselves. The primordial need to feel physical connection when illness threatens a person's intactness is again felt. Dr Gold's book helps all health care providers see the importance of this dimension of healing. Hopefully, Thai massage, like Japanese shiatsu and Chinese tui na, will become part of the new cosmopolitan approach to health care in general and body work in particular.

References

1. Leslie C 1980 Medical pluralism in world perspective. Social Science and Medicine 14B: 191–195

2. National Institutes of Health. Alternative medicine: expanding medical horizons. A report of the National Institutes of Health on alternative medical systems and practices in the United States. NIH publication no. 94-006, Washington

3. Lewith G, Aldridge D 1991 Complementary medicine and the European Community. CW Daniel, Essex

4. Ernst E, Kaptchuk T 1996 Homeopathy revisited. Archives of Internal Medicine 156: 2162–2164

5. Bhardwaj S M 1980 Medical pluralism and homeopathy: a geographic perspective. Social Science in Medicine 14B: 209–216

6. Tamulaitis C M, Auerbach G A 1992 Chiropractic growth outside of North America. In: Haldeman S (ed) Principles and practice of chiropractic. Appleton and Lange, Norwalk

7. British Medical Association 1993 Complementary medicine: new approaches to good practice. Oxford University Press, Oxford

8. Brun V, Schumacher T 1987 Traditional herbal medicine in Northern Thailand. University of California Press, Berkely

9. Golomb L 1985 An anthropology of curing in multiethnic Thailand. University of Illinois Press, Urbana

10. Sigerist H E 1951 A history of medicine, Vol 1. Oxford University Press, Oxford

Preface

Interest in the study, practice and receiving of oriental medicine and its associated techniques has seen remarkable growth in the West in the last 25 years and the terms acupuncture, t'ai Chi, shiatsu, herbal remedies, yoga and oriental massage have become part of everyday vernacular in the West. Until recently, the primary sources of these oriental imports have been China, Japan, and India. Published information on the traditional medical practices of oriental cultures has also seen tremendous growth in both quantity and quality. Curiously, however, there has been a relative lack of scholarly interest in the nation of Thailand and, in particular, its indigenous traditional medicine. The goal of this book is to begin to address this deficiency.

Archaeologists have discovered human artefacts dating from about 5000 years ago in northern Thailand, but the Thai people themselves are a more recent arrival, with the first certain historical inscription dated in the 11th century AD. By the year 1238, two Thai chieftains had rebelled against the then ruling Khmer powers and set up an independent kingdom they called Sukhothai, a Pali term that translates as 'the dawn of happiness'. Since then, an independent nation has existed in this fertile region of southeast Asia. Thailand has never been subjected to domination by a Western power. As early as 1684, the first Thai ambassador was sent to the court of the French king, Louis XIV. Thailand is currently ruled by a constitutional monarchy whose lineage dates from 1782, when the capital was relocated to Bangkok and the Ratanakosin period began.

The traditional medicine of Thailand is a distinct and comprehensive system of healing. Thai medicine traces its origins back to an historical figure, revered to this day as the 'Father Doctor', who lived in India at the same time as the historical Buddha, approximately the 5th century BC. Four branches comprise traditional Thai medicine; this book is devoted to the physical medicine, or Nuad Bo'Rarn, commonly referred to as Thai massage. The Thai word Nuad refers to touch with the purpose of imparting healing. The word Bo'Rarn, which is derived from Sanskrit, refers to something which is ancient and revered. This form of traditional body therapy has its origins in the Sangha, the monastic community that formed around the Buddha.

Thailand is over 90% Buddhist. The Wats, or monasteries, have traditionally served as the focal point of the Thai communities as centres for healing on the spiritual, emotional and physical planes. Along with Nuad Bo'Rarn, Thai medicine is composed of herbal medicines, nutritional medicines, and spiritual practices. Meditation and yoga, core components of Thai religious practice, also play an important role in Thai massage. Historically, traditional medicine has been practiced by the monks and nuns who resided in the Wats.

Thai massage differs dramatically from massage techniques as developed and practiced in the Western world:

• Thai massage is a core component of a traditional medical practice. It emphasizes pressing, compression and stretching techniques, and its treatment techniques are quite distinct from the rubbing effleurrage and petrissage techniques of Western massage. In addition, Thai massage practitioners utilize their feet, knees, elbows and forearms extensively during treatment.

• The client remains clothed in loose fitting clothing during Thai massage. No oils or other skin lubricants are utilized.

• The treatment session takes place on a pad or cotton futon that is placed on the floor or on a low platform.

• Thai massage is practiced very slowly (it is difficult to practice Thai Massage *too* slowly). A typical session can last well over 2 hours. There is an imperative that the practitioner seeks to achieve a meditative and concentrated state of mind, unencumbered by thought or fantasy, and is able to transmit this quality of mind to the client through touch.

• Finally, although it is the physical body of the client that is being addressed, the focus of treatment is primarily on the 'energy' body and on the mind. The purpose of the practice of Thai massage is to bring balance and harmony to the body, mind, and spirit of the client and thereby provide healing.

The main portion of this book (Section 2) comprises detailed photographs and step-by-step written descriptions of each technique depicted in the photographs. At first glance, many of the techniques might appear difficult to do and to receive. However, because the work is done very slowly, there is very little chance of injury. Any technique that causes pain or significant discomfort to the giver or receiver should be stopped immediately. It is essential that prior to treatment, the practitioner inquire about the client's current health, medications and medical history. Throughout the text of the book contraindications for particular procedures are listed. The practitioner must always remember that the first rule of practice is to *do no harm*.

It is my sincere hope that this book will encourage others to participate in the practice and receiving of traditional Thai massage. Furthermore, I hope that it will inspire others in professional and academic circles to further research, study, practice and write about all aspects of the traditional medicine of Thailand.

Acknowledgements

There are a number of people I wish to thank for their role in helping this book come to fruition. My parents, Harriet and Baron Gold, who instilled in me a healthy curiosity and a willingness to travel on new paths. The teachers who graciously shared their skills and knowledge. Dr Tin Yao So, my first Chinese medicine teacher, who set a spark that has never diminished. Ted Kaptchuk, teacher, friend, inspiration, who for 20 years has always helped chart new directions. Chao Khun, Therevada Buddhist monk, who introduced me to meditation in 1971. Sensei Kyoshi Kato of Osaka, Japan, who taught me Seitai Shiatsu and encouraged me to teach. The entire teaching staff, and especially Chongkol Setthakorn, at the Old Medicine Hospital, the Foundation of Shivago Komparaj in Chiang Mai, Thailand, who joyfully shared their skills, reverence, humor and touch. Waikiki Ron Rosenberger, adventurer, who led me to Chiang Mai and into my first Thai massage. Barbara Clark and the Board of Directors of the International Professional School of Bodywork (IPSB) who encouraged and helped support many phases of my work. Skip Kanester and Grey Weisheipl of IPSB who early on fell in love with Thai massage and became excellent students and teachers of the work. Jack Miller and the Boards of Directors of Pacific College of Oriental Medicine and Pacific Symposiums who helped expose Thai massage to large numbers of people through their International symposia and classrooms. Cindy Banker and the leadership of the American Oriental Bodytherapy Association who have supported the growth of Thai massage in America. Lana David, the principal model for this book, who is an excellent recipient as well as practitioner and teacher of Thai massage. Lauren Sheposh and Pnina Riter who patiently modeled for additional photographs. John and Rona Rundle of Dreamcatcher Photography whose excellent work fills these pages. Larry Emlaw whose artistic skills and over 20 years of practicing meditation made him an ideal videographer to work with during long hours of shooting and editing. My wife Pnina and daughter, Ella, who always kept the home fires burning.

Introduction: closing a circle

In December 1988, I arrived in Thailand for the first time, thereby completing an essential circle in my personal life. Seventeen years earlier, in 1971, as a 20-year-old junior pre-medical student at Oberlin College, I had my first experience in seeking mindfulness during a month-long meditation retreat led by a Theravada Buddhist monk from Thailand. This first exposure to meditation and personal growth was a profound, difficult and challenging experience for me. Primarily, I learned how far from mindfulness I was and how incessantly busy my mind was. Even so, this first experience had a lasting and influential impact on my life. Subsequent to the meditation retreat, my major at college switched from pre-medicine to religion. These studies introduced me to the spiritual literature of Eastern and Western religions.

In the first 5 years after college, from 1972 to 1977, meditation and yoga practice became a focal point of my life. During these years, I lived alone as a hermit in a log cabin on an isolated farm in rural Kentucky. My outward life revolved around physical labor in organic agriculture and forest improvement. My inner life was devoted to seeking mindfulness; seeking an ability to quiet my mind and have my mind being capable of observing 'Mind'. This inner work proved to be a very difficult and elusive task. Fortunately, I did become quite adept at organic agriculture. In addition, I loved forestry work and felt very alive and connected to nature while working amongst big trees. In fact, while I was engaged in physical labor I approached a sense of meditative mindfulness that far exceeded anything attained while seated in meditation or practicing yoga.

In the winter of 1975, I awoke one morning in my log cabin from a deep dreamspace. As my mind cleared from sleep, all I could think about was wanting to study acupuncture. The specifics of the dream never registered in my conscious mind, but the deep desire to study acupuncture never left my mind (and spirit). Up until that moment, I only had the haziest idea of what acupuncture was. There were no schools of acupuncture in America at that time. I had no role model and no personal experience of acupuncture to reference to this compulsion. Still, the seed had been planted and I set out to do whatever it took to make this dream a reality.

In the autumn of 1977, I enrolled in the New England School of Acupuncture, in Boston, Massachusetts. This was the first state approved school of acupuncture in America. My time at school in Boston was wonderful. I was a conscientious and devoted student. Upon completion of the program at the New England School, in 1979 I moved to San Diego, California and began study in a doctoral program in psychology. This course of study emphasized the emerging field of body-oriented psychology. At the time, I felt a great personal and professional need to continue my studies in healing work. Although the program at the New England School of Acupuncture was excellent, I did feel that not enough emphasis was placed on communication, emotional development and counseling skills. I therefore committed myself to advanced study in the field of psychology.

In January 1980, I received a US Embassy invitation to visit and study in the People's Republic of China, where I participated in advanced studies in Chinese medicine at Xinhua Hospital in Shanghai. This was a very important learning experience for me. Seeing and experiencing how totally integrated acupuncture, herbs, and body therapy were in the entire medical system of China was very inspiring and encouraging and my confidence and enthusiasm soared.

In 1983, I completed my doctorate in psychology and also received my license from the Medical Board of California to practice acupuncture and Chinese medicine. For the next three years, I devoted most of my time to the private practice and teaching of Chinese medicine. At this juncture of my life, I was thoroughly caught up in the activities of work and commerce, and far away from a life devoted to meditation and contemplation. By late 1985, I knew that I needed a break and a change in my day-to-day activities. I scheduled a 4-month sabbatical to travel, study, and simply 'be' in Asia. Ultimately, I traveled to Hong Kong, Taiwan, Japan and attended a week long meditation retreat in Maui on my way home. Of most significance on this journey was my apprenticeship with Shiatsu Master Kyoshi Kato in Osaka, Japan and my clinical work with Dr C. K. Butt in Hong Kong.

After my return to California, in mid-1986, I became immersed in an even busier work schedule than the one I had left: in addition to my teaching and clinical work, I helped found the Pacific College of Oriental Medicine, assumed even more teaching hours and added Board of Director responsibilities. For the next two and a half years, I worked 6 days a week. By the end of 1988, I knew I needed a significant break in my work schedule and realized that the best way for me to accomplish this was to leave the country. As I planned this sabbatical, I recognized that what I most needed was personal growth, reflection and spiritual development. Once I made this decision, the next step unfolded spontaneously. I would travel to Thailand and rekindle my study of Buddhism and meditation.

I arrived in the northern city of Chiang Mai after an all night train ride from Bangkok. It was during this initial trip to Thailand that I first experienced Traditional Thai Medical Massage. I knew I was experiencing something profound, unique and wonderful. The doing and receiving of Thai massage not only benefits the body but also facilitates a meditative experience for both giver and receiver. This potential for an experience of mindfulness is inherent in the work itself. During this very first experience of the work this glimpse of meditative mindfulness had a profound impact on me. I was hooked, and needed to further experience Thai massage. Shortly thereafter, I felt a deep desire to learn how to do the work. In one sense, the focus of my trip changed to studying medicine. But in a larger sense, I simply discovered a tool that would greatly facilitate my goals of personal and spiritual development. During the rest of my stay in Thailand, I sought out numerous practitioners in the north of the country, especially in Chiang Mai, Chiang Rai and Mae Sai. Additionally, in Bangkok, I attended tutoring sessions at Wat Pho, the site of a traditional medical school.

I returned to California in the spring of 1989 firmly committed to further study of traditional Thai medical massage. In December of 1989, I returned to Thailand. I had learned of a training program for foreigners conducted at the Old Medicine Hospital, the Foundation of Shivago Komparaj, in Chiang Mai, and had enrolled in their basic training program. I took with me a hand-held Hi-8 video camera. I was determined to record as much of the work as possible. As a teacher and practitioner of traditional Chinese medicine and Shiatsu for more than 10 years, I was struck by the scarcity of published material on the traditional medicine of Thailand; especially in comparison to the amount of literature available on Chinese medicine and Shiatsu. Also, I was not aware of any classes or academic programs in the field of Thai medicine being taught in America or Europe. Therefore, a large part of my impetus for this return trip was to gather information as a medical anthropologist. I wanted to initiate academic study in the field and work toward the development of teaching materials. This return trip to Thailand evolved into an immersion into Thai life and was one of the most wonderful experiences of my life, both personally and professionally. I lived at a simple Thai guest house, ate my meals at the local open-air marketplace and rode a bicycle alongside rice paddies on my way to and from classes. The president and instructors of the Foundation at the Old Medicine Hospital were completely cooperative in assisting me in my pursuit to learn and document the work. All the classes began and concluded with a period of chanting and meditation. The school and clinic are located down a back alley on the outskirts of Chiang Mai so that the experience of arriving for class involved taking a step deep into Thai culture.

Back once again in California in the spring of 1990, I worked to edit the hours of video material I had shot into a coherent teaching tool and to revise my lecture notes into a teaching manual that would be suitable for students in America. In conjunction with the International Professional School of Bodywork in San Diego arrangements were made to bring the primary instructor for foreigners, Chongkol Setthakorn, from the Foundation in Chiang Mai to teach at the school for 6 months. Fortunately, my enthusiasm for the work was felt by many others and a foothold for Thai massage had been established in the West.

I returned to Thailand for further study and information gathering in 1992. I also journeyed to Nepal on this trip in search of more knowledge of Ayurvedic medicine, one of the major informative influences of Thai medicine. As my own experience of and respect for Thai medicine grew, I was continually astounded by how little published material there was in the field. I had located one outstanding book, *Traditional herbal medicine in northern Thailand*, written by two Scandinavian researchers, Professor Viggo Brun and Dr Trond Schumacher.[1] Although this book has practically no information on the traditional massage, it does discuss in detail the traditional theories of Thai medicine and contains an excellent bibliography. In the summer of 1993, I traveled to Copenhagen, Denmark to meet with Professor Brun, a dedicated scholar of Thai culture and an exceptionally open and fascinating individual. I am very grateful to him for the information he provided and for the encouragement he gave me to pursue this material for publication.

Since 1990, I have been actively involved in teaching Thai massage in San Diego and at conferences and workshops around the country and overseas. Working with a professional videographer in San Diego, I completed a detailed two and a half hour teaching video of Thai massage. In cooperation with the International Professional School of Bodywork a photographic wall chart depicting many of the procedures of Thai massage was published. With every class I have taught, I have sought to improve the teaching materials and instruction available for students. All of these efforts have come together into the development of this professionally published book on Thai medical massage.

The primary goals of this book are two-fold. Firstly, I seek to provide detailed and accurate instructional guidelines for the safe and effective practice of traditional Thai medical massage (Nuad Bo'Rarn). I also hope that this book will stimulate further research, study and practical applications in the entire field of the traditional medicine of Thailand, including the herbal, nutritional, and spiritual applications, as well as the physical, massage component.

History and methods

1 Traditional Thai medicine

A brief history of medicine in Thailand

Thailand (ancient Siam) is a nation with a long and noble history stretching back hundreds of years. As with other developed Asian cultures, there has existed in Thailand for many centuries a coherent, empirically based and clinically practiced traditional medicine.

Traditional medicine in Thailand is composed of four branches: herbal medicine; nutritional medicine; spiritual practices; and manual medicine or massage (Nuad Bo'Rarn). The word Bo'Rarn is derived from the Sanskrit word Purana which is the name given to certain ancient, sacred works. Therefore, the naming of this healing work as 'ancient or sacred' means that it is derived from a body of teaching that has been handed down from generation to generation since early times and has a similar authority with the population and the Buddhist hierarchy as that of religious teachings and texts. The legendary/historical founder of Thai medicine is a native of India known as Jivaka Kumar Bhaccha (Shivago Komparaj). He is identified as a close personal associate of the historical Buddha and was the head physician of the original Sangha, the community that gathered around the Buddha. This would place him as living in India approximately 2500 years ago. The movement of medicine into Thailand accompanied the movement of Buddhist monks from India to Thailand. The precise dates of this migration are disputed, but historians place it around the 2nd century BC. What is known, is that during the reign of King Rama Khamheng (c. 1275–1317) Theravada Buddhism was made the official religion of the kingdom. Interestingly, the stone inscription from 1292 that declared Buddhism the official religion is the oldest known document written in Thai script. Little is known of other aspects of the historical development of medicine in Thailand before the mid-19th century.

For centuries, the traditional medical knowledge was transmitted orally from teacher to student in the same way as the religious texts

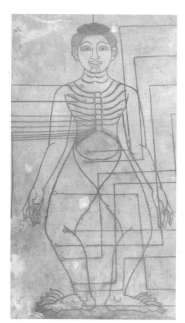

An example of one of the 60 epigraphs carved into stone by the monks at Wat Pho in 1832. These epigraphs depict the energy pathways (Sen) of the body and include explanatory notes for treatment protocols.

(sutras) of Buddhism were transmitted. The Wats, or monasteries, have always been the place where the Thai people have gone for treatment of their suffering, whether physical, emotional, or spiritual. Thai medicine in its present form developed within the context of the Buddhist community and was practiced by monks and nuns. There is mention of Nuad in a 17th-century medical scripture written on palm leaves. The medical texts were considered to be of the utmost importance and received a similar veneration to that accorded to religious texts. Many old texts were retained in the old royal capital of Ayutthia. In 1767, Ayutthia was overrun and destroyed by Burmese invaders from the north. Included in the destruction was the loss of most of the important old medical texts. In addition, most of the official records of religious, spiritual, and governmental importance to the Thai people were also destroyed.

Ancient texts on Thai medicine were mentioned as early as 1685 by Simone de la Loubère, who was a member of the embassy from the court of Louis XIV of France to the court of Siam at Ayutthia.

In 1832, the King of Siam, Rama III ordered the monks at the royal monastery in Bangkok, Phra Chetuphon Temple (commonly known today as Wat Pho), to carve epigraphs into stone depicting information that was retained in the few remaining ancient medical texts. These historically-important stone carvings were placed into the walls of the medical pavilion in the grounds of Wat Pho, where they can still be viewed by the public. They depict the energy pathways of the body and include explanatory notes describing medical treatment protocols based on therapy points located along these energy pathways (designated as Sen in Thai medicine). Altogether, there are 60 carvings at Wat Pho, with 30 depicting the front of the body and 30 the back. The carvings represent an important historical resource in Thai medicine, and their presence in the royal monastery, the most important monastery in the modern capital, indicates the reverence in which traditional medicine is held by both the royal family and the Theravada Buddhist community.

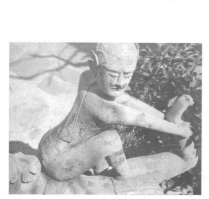

One of the carved statues in the gardens of Wat Pho, the Royal Monastery in Bangkok, that depict specific stretching techniques of Thai massage.

In recent years, there has been an increase in awareness and embracing of their traditional medicine by the Thai people. The interest of foreigners in the indigenous medicine of Thailand has also helped in this revitalization. The current monarchy of Thailand has been a strong advocate of the traditional medicine. The Crown Princess has established a foundation for the study of indigenous herbs in the treatment of cancer and HIV infection, and an organization called The Revitalization of Thai Massage, has been established to further the advancement of the study, practice, and application of traditional techniques.

Buddhist influence on Thai massage

Thai medicine has evolved within the cultural context of Theravada Buddhism and its development and history are woven into the fabric of the spiritual tenets of Buddhism. Many components of the traditional massage have been developed and utilized to facilitate seated meditation and the practice of yoga.

In Buddhist philosophy the concept of Metta is highly esteemed. Metta, which is understood as Loving Kindness, is a core component of daily life for each individual seeking awareness on the path described by the Buddha. Teachers describe Metta as the 'foundation of the world',[2] essential for the peace and happiness of oneself and others. The practice of massage and healing work is understood to be a practical application of Metta. Healing work has been closely connected to the Buddhist monasteries, Wats, of Thailand for centuries. Thai massage demonstrates the Four Divine States of mind: Loving Kindness, Compassion, Vicarious Joy, and Equanimity. In Thai Theravada Buddhism, significant emphasis is placed on the practical application of spiritual philosophy: that higher ideals should be brought into everyday life activities and decisions. The specific application of the healing techniques of Nuad Bo'Rarn is considered to be a form of meditative practice, with benefit to the recipient as well as the practitioner. The practitioner endeavors to work in a state of mindfulness, concentrated and present in each breath, each moment. Every movement, every procedure, every breath, every posture and every position is an opportunity for the practitioner and recipient to achieve clear intent and mindfulness. Working towards and in this state of awareness opens the perception and intuition of the practitioner. This allows for an acute sensitivity to subtle shifts of energy and change in the client's body and mind. This can lead to a deep therapeutic effect.

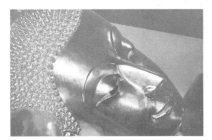

The head of a large reclining Buddha located at Wat Pho in Bangkok, the site of the traditional medical school. Buddhist influences pervade the theory, development and practice of traditional medicine in Thailand.

This philosophy and quality of touch does not rest upon nor create any dogma, nor impose any idea or specific discipline upon another human being. This quality of human exchange and awareness helps create the space and the freedom for growth and new perceptions; for the harmony, grace, and flow of universal energy that is essential for healing to occur. It is in the spirit of love and humility that the practitioner approaches the healing session. The practitioner prays for guidance and wisdom to serve at the highest levels possible. The hope is to relieve human suffering. There is no one right way to accomplish this endless task. Practitioners simply and honestly apply their skills and knowledge to the best of their abilities without attachment to the results.

Basic theories

The theories underlying traditional Thai medicine represent an interweaving of the theories, philosophies and practices of ancient India and China. Additionally, Thai medicine has evolved in the context of Theravada Buddhist culture and the monastic tradition of Thai Theravada Buddhism. The result of this historic intermingling is a purely Thai expression of medicine. According to Thai philosophy, everything in our world is made up of four elements: Earth, Water, Wind and Fire. In normal, healthy and harmonious states, the four elements exist in a dynamic, interactive balance. In situations where human beings have diseases and ailments, the elements are considered to be out of balance and the person suffers.

Another essential component of Thai medical theory describes three aspects or dynamic principles of the body to which the causes of all diseases can be traced. These three aspects, or Doshas, are the Bile (Pitta), the Wind (Vata, Lom, Feng), and the Phlegm or Mucus (Kapha). Whereas all matter known on the earth is composed of the four elements, only living matter has the Doshas. Human beings are influenced primarily by one Dosha, although aspects of all three will be present. The three Doshas have acquired a specific character from the elements that primarily influence them: Earth and Water influence Phlegm (Kapha); Fire influences Bile (Pitta); and Air influences the Wind (Vata, Lom, Feng). Kapha has the firmness and stability of Earth combined with a fluid changeability. Pitta displays the dynamic transformative energy of Fire. Vata possesses the mobility and randomness of the Wind. According to traditional theory, a person's age and the time of their life have a strong influence on the state of the three Doshas and therefore on health and disease. From birth until the age of 16 the major causative factor of disease is Phlegm (Kapha). From the age of 16 until age 32, the major causes of diseases arise from the Bile (Pitta). When an individual is age 32 and over, diseases are primarily caused by the Wind (Vata, Lom, Feng).

Drawing upon these basic theories, the aspect that most clearly relates to the practice of Thai massage is the theory of Wind.* In the practical application of the techniques of Thai massage, the slow, rhythmic presses and deep compressions are designed to affect the Wind that is present in the body. The practitioner seeks to facilitate the correct movement and placement of Wind in the body and to release the Wind from places where it has become stagnant. The numerous stretches that are a critical component of Thai massage are designed to move Wind that has accumulated in the joints of the body structure.

---

* Wind, or Feng, is also an important aspect of traditional Chinese medicine. For further reading on wind in Chinese medicine, please see references 4 and 5.

The issue of Wind

> *All functions of the body were discharged by a mysterious agency called the 'wind'. It caused the blood to flow – you could feel it in the beating pulse; the digestion to act, the bowels to move, the skin to perspire. Indigestion was from excess wind. Headaches were caused by the wind from below blowing upwards. Pains in the legs were caused by the wind from above blowing downwards. The wind (Lom) was the cause of most of the complaints from which the body suffered.*[3]

The concept of Wind is a vital theoretical component of the traditional medicines of Thailand, India, and China.[4,5] For the student and practitioner of Thai massage, a firm grasp of the qualities and issues that are ascribed to Wind is essential for effective practice and clear intention. Wind is an integral constituent of the body and a foundation element in the universe. Wind is the only aspect that is both considered as an element and also one of the three Doshas. Wind is considered the most important of the three Doshas because it sets the other two in motion and assists in the regulation of the functions of the Pitta and Kapha. When the Wind (Vata, Lom, Feng) is functioning normally, the individual has a proper regulation of all the body's activities. There will be a normalcy in the functions of digestion, assimilation and elimination. Wind provides for the guidance of mental processes and converts everything experienced by the senses into psychosomatic reactions and produces appropriate reactions. Wind initiates the desire and the will to lead an active life. Wind keeps the breathing regular, reinforces the flow of physiological activities, supports an individual's fitness for conception and promotes longevity.

According to the theories of traditional Chinese medicine, Wind (Feng) is both movement and that which generates movement in what would otherwise be still. Wind produces change and urgency in what would otherwise be slow and even. Wind arises quickly, changes rapidly and moves swiftly causing things (especially symptoms) to appear and disappear rapidly and abruptly. Wind is considered to be the primary factor in the onset of disease from external causes because the other conditions of Cold, Damp, Dry, and Heat all depend on the Wind to invade the body. In Chinese medicine, Wind also manifests as an internal factor in disease processes, usually accompanying a chronic disorder of the Liver and can contribute to symptoms such as vertigo, convulsions, migraines, hemiplegia, and vision distortion.

Many symptomologies are associated with Wind disharmony. Wind is extremely volatile and is easily influenced both in terms of quantity and quality. Wind may be in excess or be deficient in the body as a whole (leading to hyper- or hypo-functionality) or in a particular aspect or part of the body (e.g. leading to spasms, tremors, or lack of function in a limb). Wind can ascend in the body, becoming excessive in the head and causing dizziness or headaches. Wind can descend and become excessive in the legs, causing spasms. Wind tends to attack the surface of the body, causing itching, hives, and symptoms of flu, such as sneezing, cough, and runny nose. Wind can become stuck or trapped in a specific location, causing paralysis. Wind can spread anywhere in the body with the blood. Wind in conjunction with blood and lymph can become toxic and express as antisocial behavior or psychosis.

Sen: the energy pathways of the body

Thai medical theory also is based on an energetic paradigm of the body. This understanding of human life as a manifestation of universal energy is best articulated in the traditional medicine of China and is designated as Qi or Chi. In Thai medical theory, vital energy or Prana travels through the body on pathways called Sen. The Sen are closely related in theory to the meridian system of Chinese medicine. Ten primary Sen are identified. Essentially, they connect the center of the body, the abdominal region in the vicinity of the navel, to the sensory and excretory orifices. The abdominal region represents the physiological and energetic core of the body. The general location of Vata is held to be in the lower abdominal cavity. A healthy center is essential for a healthy whole person to manifest. Whereas the Sen can be correlated to the meridians of Chinese medicine, the actual naming of the Sen is more closely related to ancient India and yogic theory. The Sen names are derived from the Sanskrit language and correlates are found in the terminology associated with yogic practice. In addition to the 10 primary Sen, 72 000 Nadis are identified. The Nadis are considered the energetic network in the body where Prana (vital energy) is absorbed at the Chakras,* converted into the life energy of each of three dimensions, and distributed throughout the body/mind. The three dimensions of the body/mind are the physical body, the astral (subtle) body that is experienced as emotions, and the causal body that is expressed as intelligence and wisdom.

On the following pages are diagrams of the 10 Sen and lists of the indications that the Sen can be used to treat clinically. The lists of indications can also be understood to indicate those problems that

---

* Nadi, Prana and Chakra are specific terms from the traditions of yoga and Ayurvedic medicine of India. Chakra is used to designate centers in the body that closely correlate with the endocrine glands.

can arise when there is blockage or disharmony related to the particular Sen. Specific treatment protocols for each Sen are not included in this text. In the practical application of the work as a general massage that is outlined in this book, the Sen lines are worked on directly. The names of the Sen are listed in the Sanskrit language. Where correlations to the meridian pathways of Chinese medicine are apparent, this is duly noted.

Sen Sumana

Sen Sumana starts at the tip of the tongue, travels down the throat and chest into the solar plexus region (Ren 14). (This pathway resembles the Sushumna Nadi in the yoga tradition and part of the Conception Vessel, Ren Mai meridian in Chinese medicine.)

Indications: asthma, bronchitis, chest pain, heart diseases, spasm of the diaphragm, hiatal hernia, nausea, cold, cough, throat problems, hunger pain, diseases of the digestive system, abdominal pain, paralysis in the upper body, mania, daydreaming.

Sen Ittha

Sen Ittha starts at the left nostril, travels up inside the head and then down the throat and neck. Becomes line 1 on the back and travels

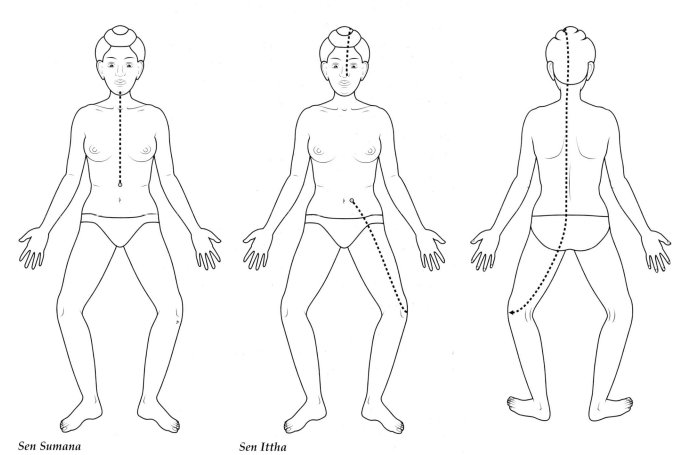

Sen Sumana   *Sen Ittha*

down the back, goes across the buttocks and continues as the 3rd outside line (lateral aspect) on the leg to the knee. At the knee, the Sen crosses to become the 1st inside line on the thigh, then ascends up the medial aspect of the leg into the abdomen and stops at the point one thumb length lateral to the navel on the left side. (Similar to the Ida Nadi in the yoga tradition and part of the Bladder meridian in Chinese medicine.)

Indications: headache, stiff neck, nose feels strange, sinus problems, cold, abdominal pain, restless legs, urinary tract disorders, back pain, knee pain.

Sen Pingkhala

This pathway is identical to Sen Ittha, only on the right side of the body. (Similar to Pingala Nadi in the yoga tradition.)

Indications: same as Sen Ittha with additions of diseases of the liver and gall bladder.

Sen Kalathari

This pathway starts at the navel and divides into two branches on the inside of the arms and two branches on the inside of the legs. The

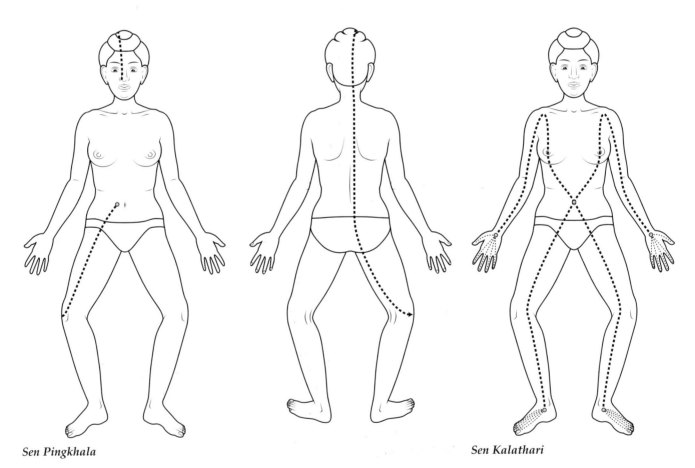

Sen Pingkhala   *Sen Kalathari*

arm branches' energy passes up from the navel through the abdominal and chest regions across the shoulders and travels down the inside middle line of the arms into the hands and crosses into the palm of the hands to the tips of all the fingers. The leg branches of the Sen travel out from the navel across the inguinal region and descend down the inside of the legs on the middle (line 2) of the leg to the foot and end at the tips of all the toes.

Indications: diseases of the digestive system, indigestion, hernia, paralysis of the arms and legs, knee pain, jaundice, whooping cough, arthritis of the fingers, chest pain, shock, rheumatic heart disease, cardiac arrhythmia, angina pectoris, sinusitis, arm and leg pain, epilepsy, schizophrenia, hysteria, mental disorders, back pain, spinal pain.

Sen Sahatsarangsi
This pathway starts in the left eye and travels inside the head through the throat and descends down the left side of the chest and abdomen. It continues to the outside of the leg and descends along the 1st line of the outer leg into the foot, then crosses the foot and ascends up the inside of the leg along line 1, and crosses the inguinal area and ends just below the navel. (This line corresponds in part to the Stomach meridian in acupuncture.)

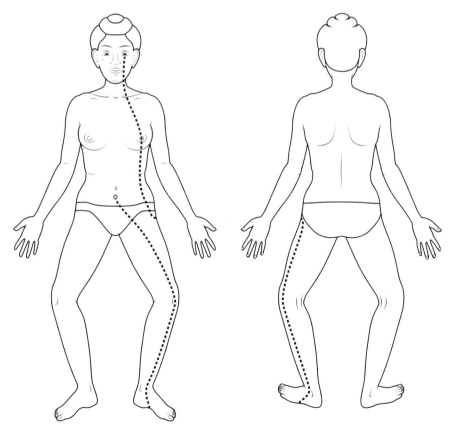

Sen Sahatsarangsi

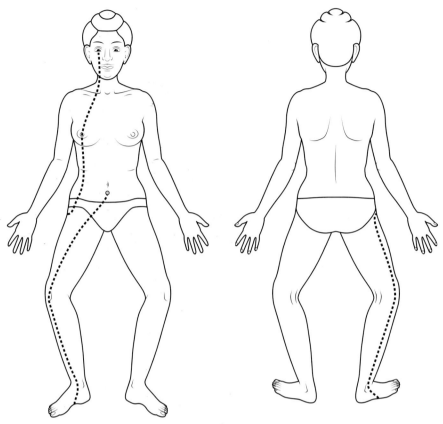

Sen Thawari

Indications: facial paralysis, toothache, throat pain, red and swollen eye, cataract, impaired eye function, fever, chest pain, manic depression, gastrointestinal disease, urogenital diseases, leg paralysis, knee joint pain, numbness of leg, hernia.

Sen Thawari
This pathway begins at the right eye and then follows the same course as Sen Sahatsarangsi, but on the right side of the body.

Indications: same as Sen Sahatsarangsi with additions of jaundice and appendicitis.

Sen Lawusang
This pathway starts in the left ear and travels down the left side of the throat into the chest toward the left nipple. At the nipple, the line turns inward and travels toward the navel and ends above the navel in the solar plexus region.

Indications: deafness, ear diseases, tinnitus, cough, facial paralysis, toothache, chest pain, gastrointestinal disorders.

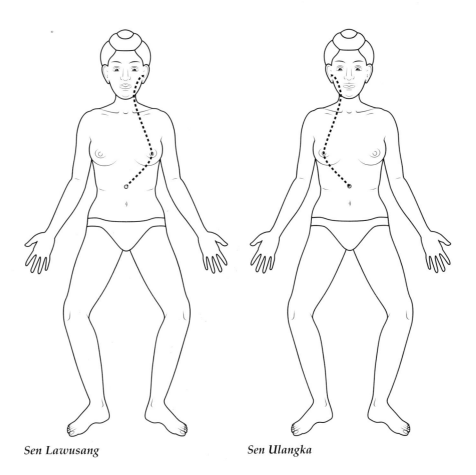

Sen Lawusang   *Sen Ulangka*

Sen Ulangka

This pathway begins in the right ear and follows the same path as Sen Lawusang but on the right side of the body, ending above the navel.

Indications: same as Sen Lawusang with additions of insomnia, itching under the skin.

Sen Nanthakrawat

Sen Nanthakrawat comprises two lines:

a starts at the navel, descends through the urethra and ends at the urine passageway. This is called Sen Sikhini.

b starts at the navel and descends through the colon to join the anus. This is called Sen Sukhumang.

Indications: hernia, frequent urination, female infertility, impotence, premature ejaculation, irregular menstruation, uterine bleeding, urinary retention, diarrhoea, abdominal pain.

Sen Khitchanna
This pathway runs from the navel to the penis in men and is known as Sen Pitakun; in women it is known as Sen Kitcha, running from the navel through the uterus into the vagina.

Indications: same as with Sen Nanthakrawat, including balancing libido.

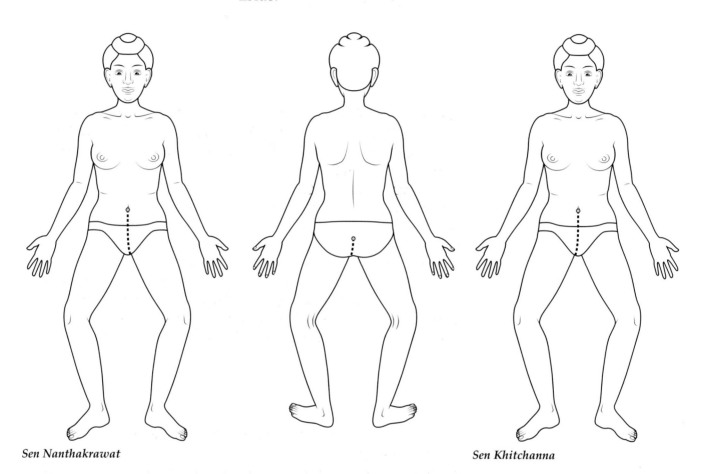

Sen Nanthakrawat   *Sen Khitchanna*

2 Rules, methods and techniques

The instructional information in this book is based on the program taught in Chiang Mai at the Old Medicine Hospital, the Foundation of Shivago Komparaj. This is considered a northern style of Thai massage. The training program at the Foundation of Shivago Komparaj is conducted in a traditional manner. A ritual prayer in the Pali language is chanted in veneration of the Father Doctor twice daily. This ceremony, called Wai Khru, is offered as a mark of respect to our teachers and in the hope that the studies and practice will lead to good conduct and action, and lessening of human suffering. A fuller description of the ceremony, including the text of the mantra, appears in the Appendix (page 201). Specific rules and methods of Thai massage are outlined for students to learn and to follow. In the following sections, I have expanded and added explanations to the information as presented at the Old Medicine Hospital.

Rules

1. The student must study diligently the techniques and practice of Thai massage.
2. Thai massage is not to be practiced in public places, such as the market places. This rule is meant to distinguish the Wats, or monasteries, and healing clinics from the market place. The Wats are the place where Thai people go for nourishment of the spirit, mind and body and to express devotion. The Wats are not places of commerce.
3. The practitioner should not hope for any gains. Historically, the monks and nuns performed this work. The practice of healing work is an expression of 'Metta', or Loving Kindness. The practice is its own reward.
4. A practitioner should never take patients from another doctor nor speak unkindly of another doctor.
5. Practitioners should never boast about their knowledge. There is always someone else who knows more than you do. The quest for

knowledge of human health and illness is endless. There is always more that is unknown than known. Human suffering is without limits. Practitioners should approach each individual case with humility and gratitude to their teachers

6. All practitioners, students, and teachers need to ask for advice and listen to people who know more than they do.

7. Students and practitioners should bring a good reputation to their schools and teachers. This is accomplished by adherence to the other rules outlined.

8. Certificates of study and accomplishment in Thai massage should only be given to qualified individuals.

9. Students, teachers, and practitioners should give thanks and appreciation everyday to the Father Doctor.

Methods

1. Practitioners work in a meditative and concentrated state of mind. They endeavor to work in a state of mindfulness: concentrating and fully present in each moment. Practitioners seek to focus their thoughts and intentions to the purpose of the treatment. They maintain a focus on their breathing. Random thoughts and ideas are to be seen for what they are, and then attention is re-focused on the healing work at hand.

2. Prior to the application of therapy, practitioners must ask clients about their current and past state of health. They should keep a written chart for each client, noting the health history, current complaints, and response to previous treatments. Any illness, use of medications or herbs or operations must be noted. Particular attention must be given to any client with a history of heart disease, high blood pressure, varicose veins or problems with blood clotting. The practitioner must know if a woman is pregnant or having her monthly menstruation. The practitioner encourages the client to give feedback during the treatment session as to how they are feeling. The client is requested to let the practitioner know if any procedure causes discomfort and if the pressure of treatment is either too deep or too soft.

3. The techniques of Thai massage are applied very slowly. Students should remember that it is difficult to work too slowly. Although on first viewing many of the techniques appear difficult to give and to receive, this is not necessarily accurate. By working slowly, practitioners can be acutely aware of a client's state of receptivity. When practitioners reach the limit of their client's ability to accept a procedure, they will know it immediately. Because practitioners are working very slowly and in a state of heightened awareness, there is very minimal danger of injury.

4. The palm pressing technique is considered an integrative technique to be utilized before and after the detailed work (e.g. treating the Sen lines of the legs) of thumb pressing has been applied. Thai massage has no long stroking techniques, such as the effleurage technique of Western-style massage. Effleurage is utilized in massage for working large areas, especially after more detailed work has been applied. In Western massage, this is considered an integrative technique.

5. After a point has been treated directly with either thumb or finger pressure, the practitioner works the area in a circular motion with thumb, finger or palm circles.

6. The stop the blood flow technique in the groin and armpit area is never utilized in cases of high blood pressure, heart disease, or varicose veins. The rationale for the application of the stop the blood flow techniques stems from the origins of this style of treatment in the monastic communities. Throughout history, this treatment has been utilized to facilitate meditation and yoga practice. Monks are able to sit cross-legged for hours and then stand up without pain or the discomfort from having their legs 'fall asleep'. They can accomplish this seemingly impossible task because they have developed the ability to move their blood flow through deeper passageways. The stop the blood flow techniques enhance the movement of blood through these deeper circulatory passageways.

7. Practitioners must work with proper body mechanics. There is a potential for injury if practitioners do not work with proper body mechanics. At no time should practitioners carry out a procedure that causes pain in their own body. Ideally, they become aware of their own energy center, an area located in the core of their body about 3 inches below the navel. All movement originates in this core area below the navel. The strength of the pressure in the hands and fingers comes from the weight of the body that travels down straight arms. Practitioners learn to conserve their own energy by working in a rocking motion. Students and practitioners are strongly advised to receive regular Thai massage and also to practice yoga, stretching, and meditation. The Chinese practices of Qi Kong and T'ai Chi are excellent techniques for becoming aware of and moving from the energy center (called the T'an T'ien) area below the navel.

8. The practitioner never presses directly down onto the knees or the other joints and bones of the client's body. Circular motion techniques with the fingers, thumbs, or palms are used over the knees, joints and along the bones.

9. When the thumb is utilized for direct downward pressure, the ball of the thumb, not the tip is used.

10. Abdominal massage is a very important component of this system of treatment. According to Thai medical theory, all of the vital Sen line energy originates deep in the abdomen in the vicinity of the navel. Abdominal massage is never given within 1 hour of the completion of a meal.

11. Cleanliness and hygiene are important. Practitioners must clean their own hands and feet prior to the healing session. The area where treatment is to be given must be clean and orderly. Also, the client should be clean.

12. Before the start of the treatment, practitioners should take a moment to quiet their mind, give thanks to the Father Doctor, and pray that good come from the treatment. Om Namo . . .

Techniques

The clinical application of Thai massage utilizes a variety of treatment techniques. The following are descriptions of the techniques that are used and prescribed in Section 2 (practical application).

Palm press (PP)

The entire palmar surface of the hand is evenly used, creating a direct downward vector into the client's body. The practitioner works with straight arms and uses shifting body weight to direct the pressure. Care must be made to not emphasize the heel of the hand nor to knead with the fingers. The palm press procedure is designated as the integration technique that is utilized after detailed thumb and

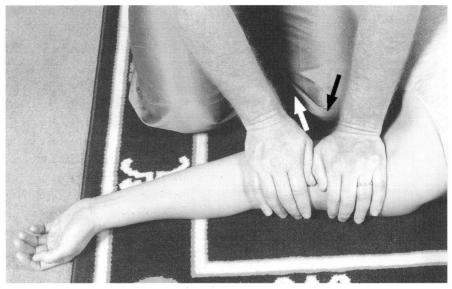

Palm press

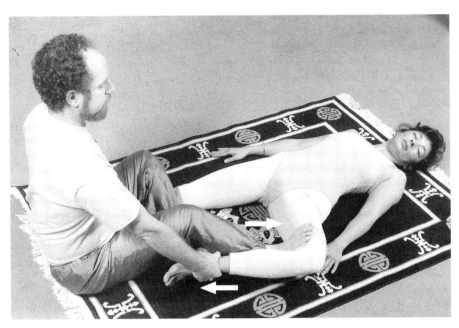

Foot press

finger work has been applied. Palm presses are done with both hands working simultaneously or alternatively. Walking-palm presses, e.g. working from the feet up and down the legs or from the upper back to the sacrum, is an application of the technique that is frequently utilized.

Foot press (FP)

The sole of the foot is utilized to deliver a firm compression to the client's body. The technique begins with the practitioner's leg bent and foot in direct contact with the client's body (e.g. the medial thigh muscles). As the practitioner's leg straightens, the thrust of the pressure is applied by the foot. The foot press is usually accompanied by a counter-force of pulling with the hand at the ankle. Care must be taken to not use the heel of the foot nor to apply excessive pressure.

Thumb press (TP)

The ball of the thumb is utilized to exert a direct downward vector. The point or tip of the thumb is not used. Thumb presses are used to treat along the Sen energy lines and into muscles. The thumbs deliver pressure that is generated from the abdominal core of the practitioner and travels down the straight arms into the hands. Use of the thumbs by exerting force in the arms and hands can quickly lead to fatigue and discomfort. Often the thumbs work in a pattern/sequence of 'thumb-chasing-thumb but never catching'. In this pattern, one thumb moves into the body as the other thumb lifts out, in a piston-like movement.

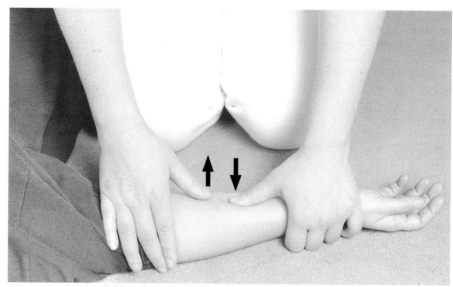

Thumb press

Elbow press (EP)

The elbow is used to treat points on the bottom of the feet. The elbow is placed on the point and the practitioner's weight is pressed down into the elbow. The elbow pressure is released by bringing the forearm forward. The practitioner never simply lifts the elbow off the point.

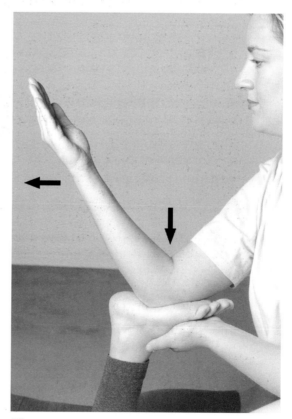

Elbow press

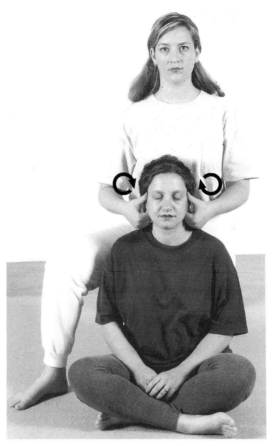

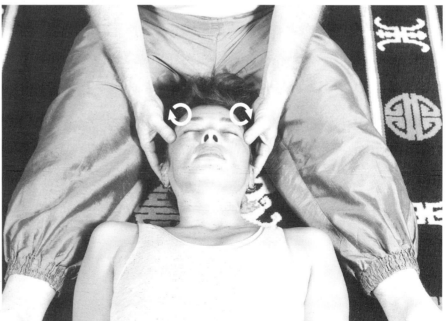

Thumb circle

Thumb circle (TC)

Circular movements of the thumbs are used on the face, head, hands and feet. Thumb circles are utilized over bones, because the practitioner never presses directly down onto bones.

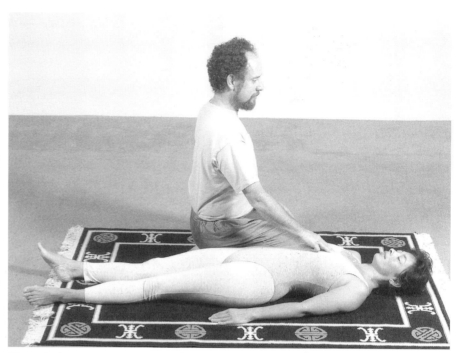

Finger circle

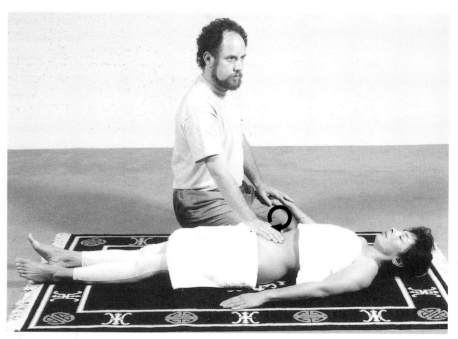

Palm circle

Finger circle (FC)

The tips of the finger(s), usually the three middle fingers are utilized together in a circular motion. This technique is used over the sternum, below the clavicle, in the intercostal spaces, along the edges of the scapula and on the face.

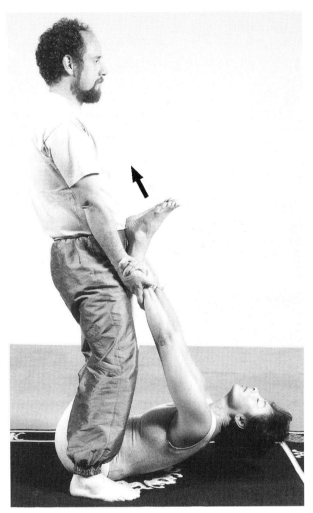

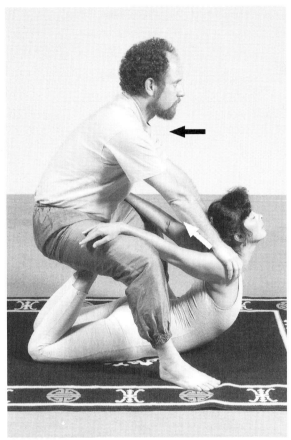

Stretching

Palm circles (PC)

Slow circular movements are made with the entire palmar surface, including the heel of the hand and fingers. Palm circles are used extensively as an integrative procedure with deep abdominal treatment.

Stretching

A critical component of Thai massage is stretching of the limbs, torso and neck. The stretching procedures are made by creating a force/counter-force in various locations of the body. As an example, the practitioner pulls at the ankle while simultaneously pressing with the foot into the client's medial thigh. The stretches create elongation and expansion, and open up the joint spaces. The practitioner seeks to give the client an expanded sense of his or her body. With the utilization of the stretches, the goal of working very slowly is especially vital. The practitioner must sense the holding patterns in the client's body and never forcibly stretch the client beyond what is comfortable.

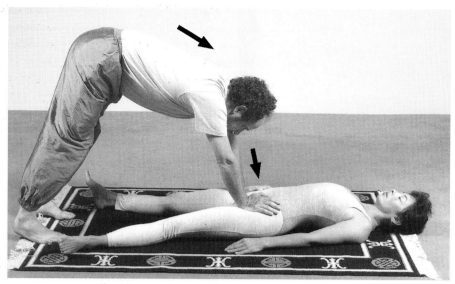

Stopping the blood flow

Stopping the blood flow
On the femoral artery in the inguinal groove and on the axillary artery in the axilla, the practitioner locates the pulse and exerts a deep downward pressure with the heel of the hand in order to obstruct the superficial flow of the blood. The practitioner retains the pressure for up to 30 seconds. This technique is never used on clients with a history of circulatory problems, or on those taking medication for the heart or circulation. The purpose of this technique is to force the blood flow into deeper circulatory patterns. Additionally, this technique is believed to stimulate the flow of Prana energy. The Thai technical term for this procedure is Perd Pra-Too Lom, meaning, Opening the Gate of the Wind. This is especially important for individuals who spend long periods of time in a cross-legged meditation postures.

The stopping of the blood flow is absolutely contraindicated with clients with heart problems and circulatory problems, including varicose veins.

Precautions and contraindications

'Above all else, do no harm'

The techniques presented in this book comprise the physical medicine of traditional Thai medical practice. Throughout the history of Thailand, these techniques have been utilized to treat the wide array of complaints that afflict mankind, including problems of internal medicine as well as structural and neurological complaints. Additionally, for many centuries Thai medicine has addressed problems of a psychological and spiritual nature. As with any medical practice, traditional or modern, there are certain basic criteria that must be met before practical application commences. The practitioner must have a clear understanding of the problem(s) to be addressed. The practitioner must learn of any previous surgeries, current usage of medications, and any precautions advised by the client's medical doctor. The practitioner must have a treatment plan and specific goals which he or she seeks to accomplish in treatment. In addition, care and caution must always be exercised in treatment.

The nature of Thai massage demands that the practitioner be especially attentive to precautions in treatment and be very clear as to any pre-existing problems the client might have which would require that certain procedures be eliminated from the treatment protocol. The following guidelines should be followed:

- Thai massage treatment is conventionally contraindicated in the treatment of cancer.

- Clients who are very ill and in a weakened state should not be treated.

- If there is high fever, treatment should not be given.

- Clients who suffer from osteoporosis should be treated with great caution with the stretching procedures and only with very light pressure.

- Clients who bruise quite easily and who are taking blood thinning medication should be treated with only a very light pressure.

- Clients who are experiencing acute pain along the spine should not receive any procedures that worsen the pain and the stretches with the client in a prone position should be eliminated.

- If the client has previously had surgery on the spine (such as a laminectomy), all stretches in a prone position where the legs are raised are eliminated.

- Clients who are pregnant should be treated with caution. There should be no abdominal work nor pressure on the low back. The best approach for treatment of a pregnant woman is to work with the client in a lateral recumbent position.

- In Thailand, women are not treated during menses. This is a cultural taboo and not a medical precaution.

- The procedures known as 'stopping the blood flow' are eliminated in treating clients with a history of heart problems, diabetes, and vascular problems.

There are specific localized problems that need to be noted and avoided during treatment. These include:

- fractures

- varicose veins

- wounds and bruises
- inflammation of joints and/or skin lesions
- abdominal area less than 1 hour after a meal.

In Section 2 (Practical application), where the procedures are described in detail, specific precautions are listed where appropriate and highlighted by the symbol illustrated here (left). At all times, the practitioner must remember that 'if in doubt, leave it out'. Additionally, the practitioner must always recognize that it is his or her responsibility to question clients in great detail about their medical history. The practitioner seeks to work with heightened awareness and sensitivity. The practitioner always encourages clients to speak up during the massage if they require a deeper or softer touch or if they are experiencing discomfort.

Practical application

3 Client in supine position

Legs and feet

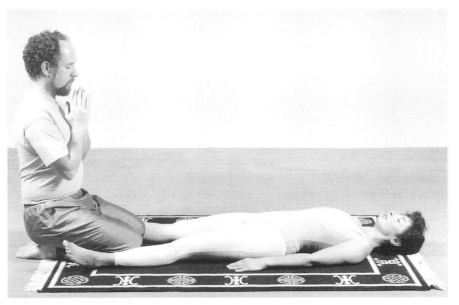

Fig. 1

1. Kneel at the feet of the client. Take a moment, with your palms touching, to quiet and focus your thoughts, seeking to create a harmony and balance within yourself before you begin the treatment. In your mind, give thanks to the Father Doctor and request that the client be released from illness, stress and pain and that there be a positive outcome to the treatment.

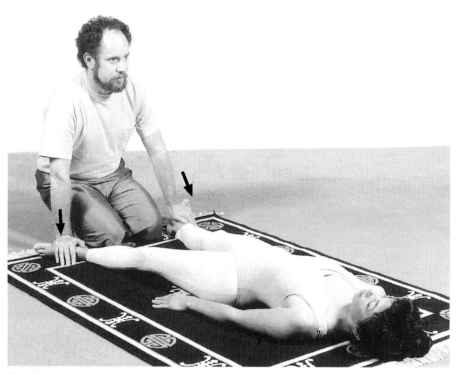

Fig. 2A

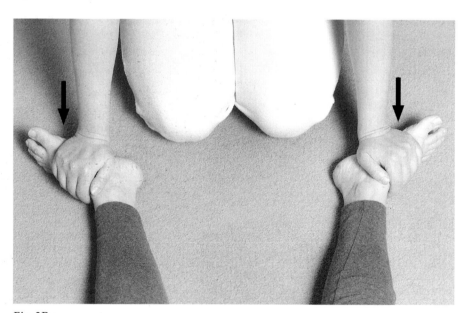

Fig. 2B

2. Palm press the medial aspect of the feet. Keep your elbows straight, rocking from side to side, working along the medial arch of the entire foot. Repeat the palm presses many times.

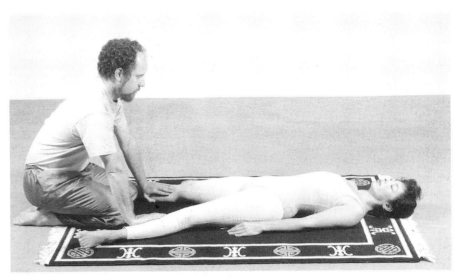

Fig. 3A

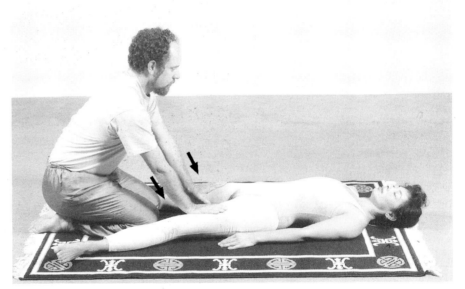

Fig. 3B

3. Continue with walking palm presses up and back down the entire medial aspect of the legs from the feet to the inguinal crease. At the knees, there is no direct palm pressure. The hand is cupped over the patella and gentle circular movements are made. Repeat the walking palm presses up and down the legs as many times as desired.

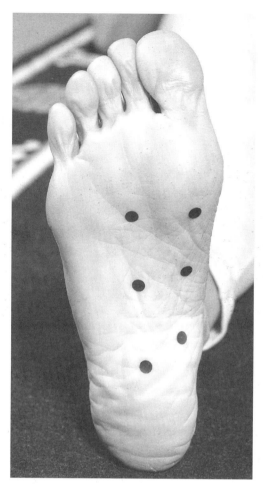

Fig. 4A

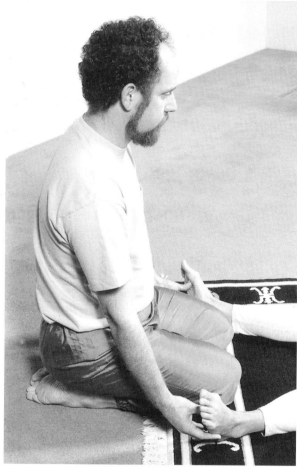

Fig. 4B

4. Six point locations are identified on the bottom of the foot. Point 1 is just posterior to the ball of the foot on the center line directly below the middle toe; point 2 is approximately an inch posterior to point 1; and point 3 is an inch posterior to point 2, directly in front of the heel (calcaneous bone).

Working on both feet simultaneously, thumb press into points 1. Hold each thumb press for approximately 5–10 seconds and release slowly. Then press points 2 and 3.

Point 4 is located by moving medially approximately an inch from point 3; point 5 is superior to point 4; and point 6 is directly behind the metatarsals in line with the big toe medial to point 1.

Press each point on both feet, working points 1 through 6 sequentially.

This pattern can be followed just once or repeated three times, with moderate pressure the first time, firmer pressure the second time and again with a moderate pressure the third time. After completion of the direct presses into the points on the bottom of the foot, use the palm presses on the medial aspect of the feet for integration.

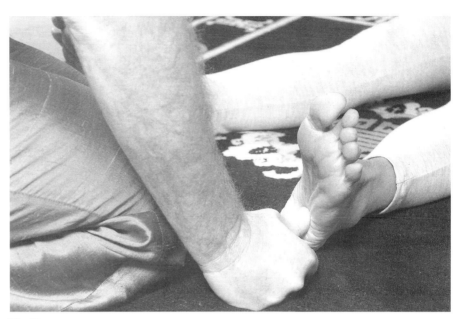

Fig. 5

5. Five lines on the soles of both feet are identified. Each line begins at point 3 (see above), which is located just in front of the heel (the calcaneous bone).

Thumb press from point 3 in a direct line towards the big toe.

At the ball of the foot where the metatarsal bones are located, stop the thumb presses and change to small thumb circles. Continue with thumb circles across the ball of the foot and along the big toe. At the end of the toe, squeeze and press the tip of the toe.

Return to point 3 just in front of the calcaneous at the heel and resume thumb presses through the soft part of the foot up to the metatarsal bones in line with the second toe. Proceed with thumb circles along the second toe, pull and press at the tip of the toe, and return to the heel point 3.

Repeat this procedure for the next three toes, working both feet simultaneously. Upon completion of this procedure for all five toes on both feet, use palm presses on the feet for integration.

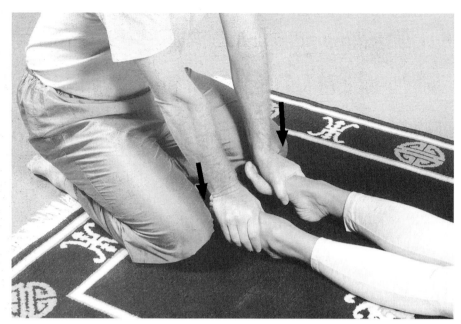

Fig. 6A

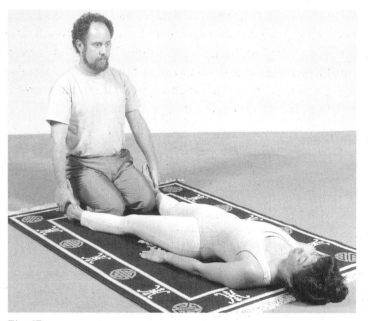

Fig. 6B

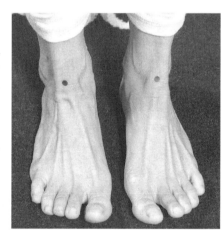

Fig. 6C

6. Palm press down along the top of the feet, stretching both the feet and the ankles. The feet are kept in line with the legs so that there will be an extension of the tendons of the foot and ankle. The first palm press is just in front of the ankle; the second in the middle of the foot over the arch; the third palm press is over the toes.

Palm press back from toes to ankles in a sequential movement pattern in position 1, 2, 3, 2, 1. The depth of pressure is varied from moderate, to deep, to moderate.

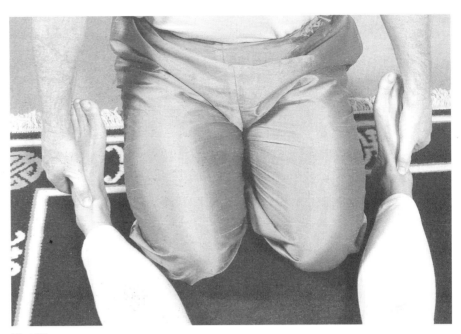

Fig. 6D

Thumb press into the hollow at the center of the top of the ankle between the tendons of extensor digitorum longus and hallicus longus (the acupoint Stomach 41 Jiexi). The fingers are wrapped around the lateral side of the foot on the little toe side. The foot is pronated toward the head, keeping the ankle on the ground. Hold the thumb press for approximately 5 seconds.

Continue with thumb circles down the groove between the first and second toes until reaching the phalangeal bones of the toes. At the toes, make thumb circles along the big toes. At the end of the toes, give a gentle pinch, a pull and then slide off.

Return to the hollow at the top of the foot and thumb press at the acupoint Stomach 41 Jiexi. Release the press and continue with thumb circles between the second and third toes and then thumb circle out the second toe, finishing with a pinch and a pull at the toes.

This pattern is continued with the thumb presses followed by thumb circles to the third and fourth toes.

To treat the little toe, make finger circles along the lateral side of each foot using the middle fingers of each hand, and then thumb circles out the little toe and finally pinch and pull the little toes. Integrate these detailed procedures with alternating palm presses on both feet.

Starting just in front of the heel along the medial arch between the pink and white skin, thumb press just underneath the bone. Continue with three or four thumb presses going out along the arch from the heel toward the junction of the metatarsal bones.

After the thumb presses that were moving in a distal direction, thumb press back towards the heel and then integrate with palm presses.

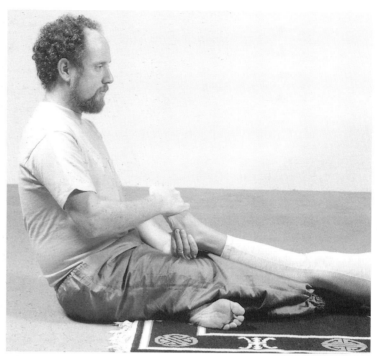

Fig. 7A

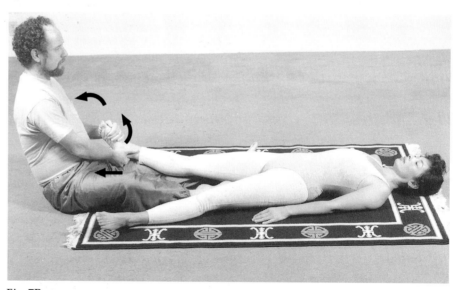

Fig. 7B

7. (Procedures 7, 8 and 9 are carried out on one foot at a time.) Sit at the client's feet, with your outside leg extended straight and the client's leg resting on the thigh of the straight leg. Hold the client's foot with the heel resting in the palm of the hand. With the other hand, hold in the vicinity of the toes. Make full circular rotations of the foot from the ankle, five times clockwise and five times counter-clockwise. Repeat the rotations three times. With each rotation, lean back slightly, stretching the foot and ankle. The client will feel the stretch into their hip joint.

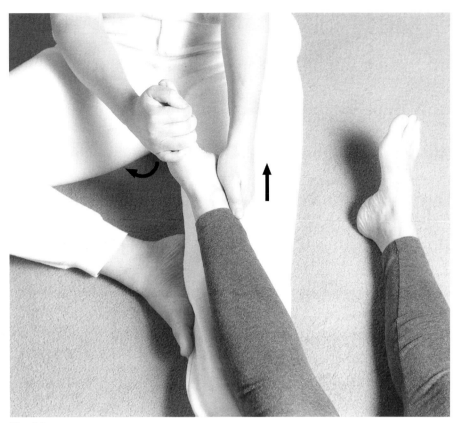

Fig. 8A

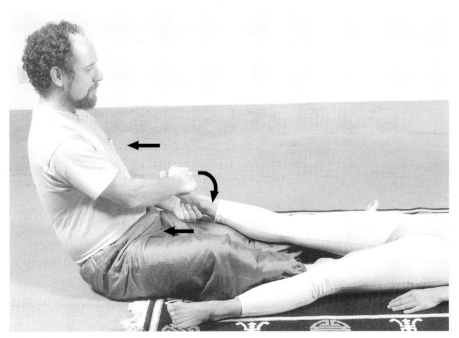

Fig. 8B

8. Grasp the foot across the medial arch, lean back and twist the foot laterally. Repeat the movements from the arch to the toes and back to the arch in a pattern, 1, 2, 3, 2, 1.

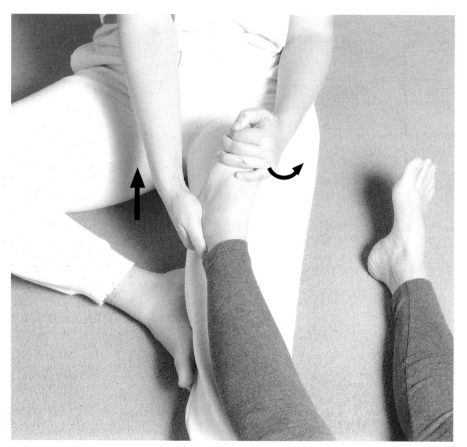

Fig. 8C

Switch hands and repeat the grasping, stretching and twisting, but now rotating medially.

Repeat the stretch and twist in a pattern of 1, 2, 3, 2, 1, moving distally and then proximally.

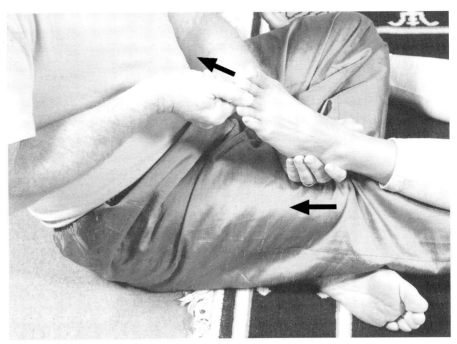

Fig. 9

9. Hold the heel of the foot in one hand and with the other hand work one toe at a time. Rotate each toe individually with the purpose of relaxing and loosening the joint. Hold firmly at the toe, lean back and give a slight pull, possibly creating a cracking or a popping sound.

Repeat for each toe and follow with gentle kneading and palm pressing into the foot for relaxation.

Complete procedure 9, go back to procedure 7, and carry out the procedures on the other foot.

10. Place the heels of the feet side by side and palm press the top of the feet, moving from the ankle out to the toes, working positions 1, 2, 3, 2, 1. Vary the pressure from soft to medium to firmer, ending with a soft press. (See illustration 6A.)

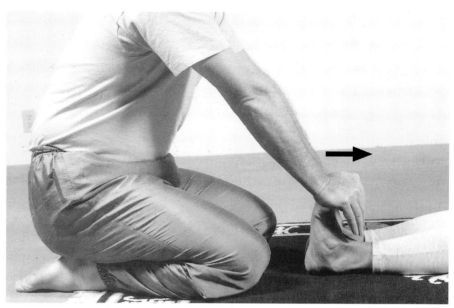

Fig. 11A

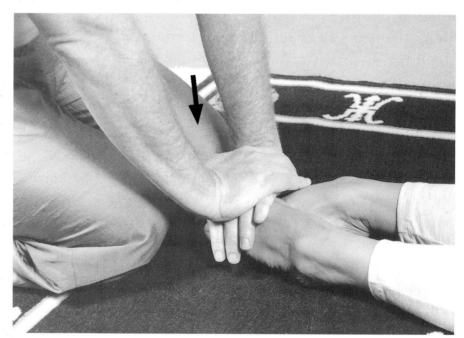

Fig. 11B

11. Keep the heels close together, grasp across the toes, the heel of the hands against the arch, and press the toes toward the head. This procedure will create an extension of the Achilles tendon. Repeat this three times with the first press done softly, the second time firmly and the third time softly.

Place the left foot over the right foot. Put both of your hands on top of the feet, palm on palm, and press down three times, creating a stretch and elongation.

Cross the feet in a reverse pattern, with the right on top of left, and repeat the presses three times.

Following the presses, separate the feet and do alternating palm presses on the feet, then walking palm presses up and down the legs, completing the first section of the massage.

Working the (Sen) lines of the legs

This section of treatment is on the (Sen) lines on the medial and lateral aspects of the lower and upper legs. The technique utilized for treating the lines of the legs is thumb presses in the pattern of 'thumb-chasing-thumb but never catching'. This is done very slowly. A piston-like pattern with the thumbs is created. Place both thumbs on the skin, with a space left open between the thumbs. As the right thumb presses in, the left thumb is released. Then as the left thumb presses in, the downward movement will release the right thumb. The right thumb then presses in at the space that was open between the thumbs and the left thumb releases. This pattern is repeated up and down the (Sen) lines.

The locations where the three lines on the medial leg begin are in the vicinity of the medial malleolus. The first point is just below the tip of the medial malleolus at the acupoint Kidney 6 Zhaohai. The second line begins midway between the medial malleolus and the Achilles tendon in the hollow at the acupoint Kidney 3 Taixi. The third line begins just medial to the Achilles tendon. The lines then follow the contour of the leg, up the lower leg to the vicinity of the knee.

Above the knee, the thigh is much wider so that the distance between the lines is greater. The first line continues at the medial superior border of the patella and then traces up the abductors to the inguinal crease. The second line continues from in the hollow posterior to the first line, travels up the middle of the abductor region, and ends in the inguinal region at the site of the pulsing of the femoral artery. Line 3 continues from adjacent to the tendon of semitendinosus. It runs parallel to line 2 up into the inguinal area in the vicinity of the groin.

The first line on the lateral aspect of the leg begins anterior and inferior to the lateral malleolus in the hollow at the point Gallbladder 40 Qiuxu and continues up the lower leg, one finger breadth lateral to the crest of the tibia. Line 2 begins just below the lateral malleolus at the acupoint Urinary Bladder 62 Shenmai and runs up the lower leg on a line between the tibia and fibula bones. Line 3 begins in the hollow between the lateral malleolus and the Achilles tendon, at the acupoint Urinary Bladder 60 Kunlun and continues up the lower leg along the posterior border of the fibula.

Above the knee, line 1 continues at the lateral superior border of the patella and follows along superior to the iliotibial tract, ending anterior to the iliac spine. Line 2 comes up the middle of the iliotibial tract, across the tensor fascia lata, and ends just below the superior aspect of the iliac spine. Line 3 begins just superior to the attachment of the tendon of the iliotibial tract at the knee, continues along the posterior border of the iliotibial tract, and ends in the gluteal region.

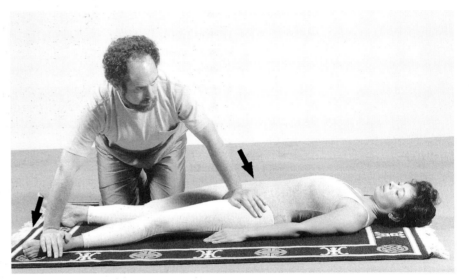

Fig. 12

12. Move to the side of the client. Reach across the closest leg and hold the other leg at the ankle with one hand and on the anterior iliac spine with the other hand; stretch the entire leg.

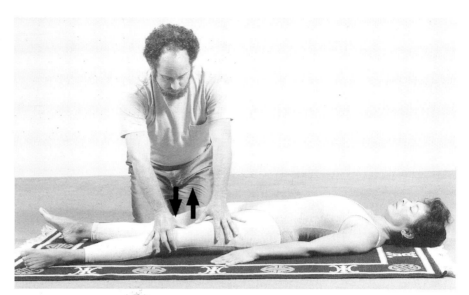

Fig. 13A

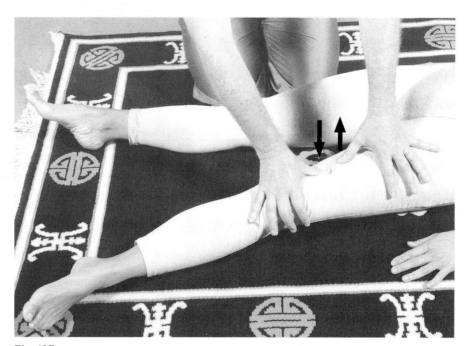

Fig. 13B

13. Palm press with the superior hand down from the hip to the knee and with the hand at the ankle, palm press up toward the knee. When the hands meet in the vicinity of the knee, continue with alternate palm presses up and then down the medial aspect of the entire leg.

Begin thumb-chasing-thumb technique up line 1. Work up line 1, down line 1; up line 2, down line 2; up line 3, down line 3. Upon completion of line 3, integrate the entire medial leg with palm presses.

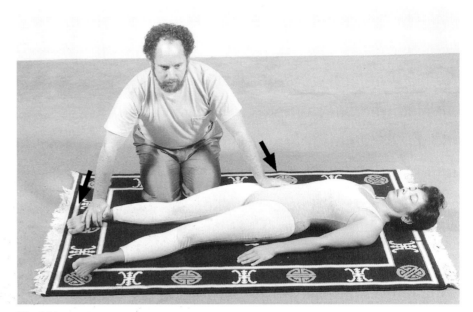

Fig. 14A

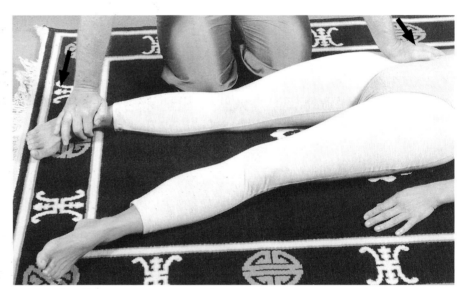

Fig. 14B

14. Remain seated in the same position to begin treatment of the lateral aspect of the closest leg. Hold at the ankle and at the iliac spine and stretch the entire leg. Palm press from the hip to the knee with one hand and from the ankle to the knee with the other hand. Continue with palm presses up and down the entire lateral aspect of the leg.

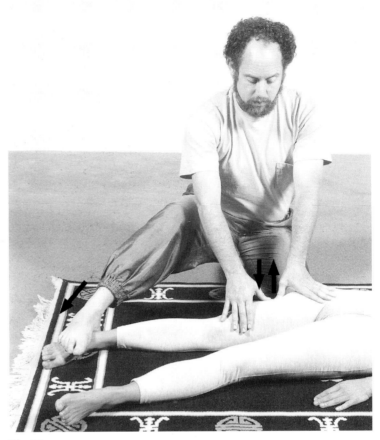

Fig. 15

15. Utilizing the thumb-chasing-thumb technique, work up and down line 1; then, up and down line 2; and finally up and down line 3. Upon completion of the thumb work on the three lines, palm press the entire leg for integration.

Sit at the other side of the client. Repeat all the procedures (the stretch, palm presses, thumb-chasing-thumb, and palm presses) on the second leg. First the medial aspect of the leg is treated, followed by the lateral aspect of the other leg. Place your foot at the client's ankle to rotate and hold the client's leg to facilitate access to line 3.

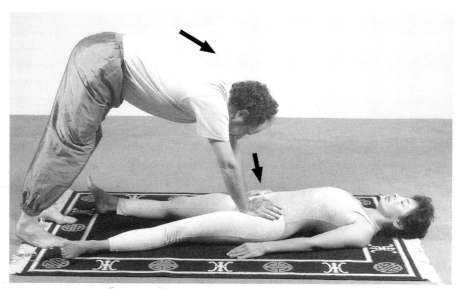

Fig. 16

16. Upon completion of the leg lines, move and kneel at the client's feet. Work both legs with walking palm presses.

At the inguinal crease, check for the pulse of the femoral artery, located at the end of line 2 on the medial thigh, (having previously checked that the client: has no history of cardiac problems; no circulatory problems; no pace-maker; no medication is being used to thin the blood; is not pregnant; does not have varicose veins in the legs).

Place the heels of your hands over the pulsing femoral artery. Slowly and skilfully, obstruct the artery with downward pressure, lifting your entire body up and bringing your weight forward into your hands. Hold this position for 30–60 seconds. Then lower your body very slowly back into a kneeling position and slowly release the pressure in heels of the hands.

Wait several seconds, allowing the blood flow to return to a normal pattern, and then palm press back down to the feet.

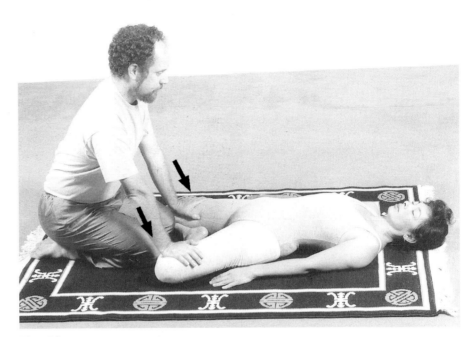

Fig. 17A

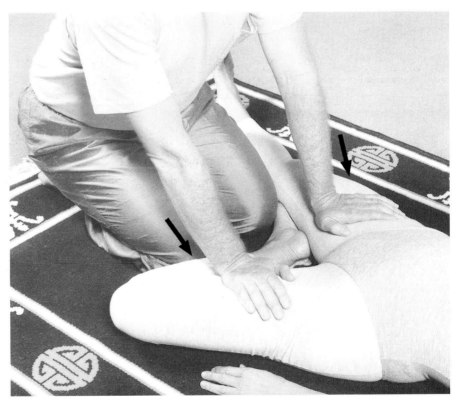

Fig. 17B

17. Bend the client's leg, placing the foot of the bent leg in the vicinity of the knee of the client's straight leg. Palm press on the thighs of both legs.

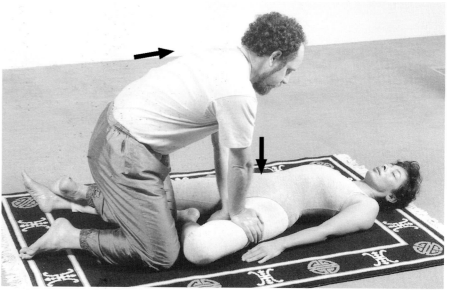

Fig. 18A

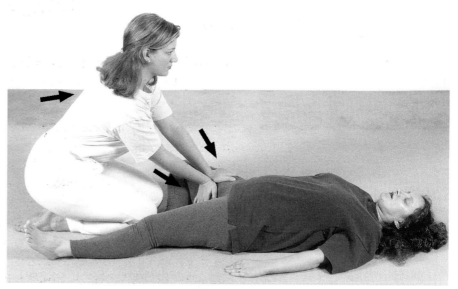

Fig. 18B

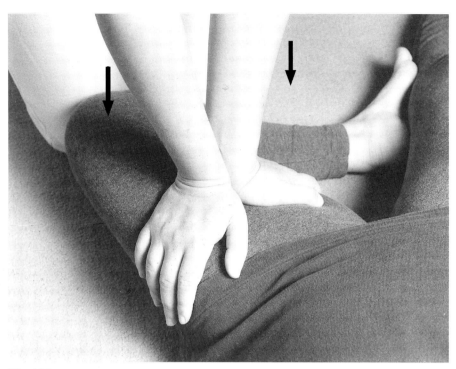

Fig. 18C

18. Shift both hands to the bent leg and palm press on the thigh down to the knee with one hand and from the foot to the knee with the other hand.

Bring the hands together just above the knee and proceed with palm presses from the knee working proximal to the inguinal area and back down toward the knee. Palm press in the pattern at positions 1, 2, 3, 2, 1 ending up just superior to the knee.

Treatment pattern 1, 2, 3, 2, 1 explained
At numerous places in the text you are instructed to work at positions 1, 2, 3, 2, 1. This directs you to initiate work in an area, for example, the medial thigh close to the knee, and to consider that area as position 1. Position 2 is just proximal to position 1, and position 3 is proximal to position 2. After working in position 3, move distally back to position 2 and finally back to position 1. This pattern of 1, 2, 3, 2, 1 creates a flow and a rhythm to the work which is both effective therapeutically and very comfortable for the client.

A variation of the technique allows you to vary pressure in a patterned manner. Working proximally, treat position 1 with moderate pressure, then treat position 2 with a deeper pressure, and then position 3 again with a lighter pressure. Moving distally, treat position 2 deeply and then position 1 with a lighter touch.

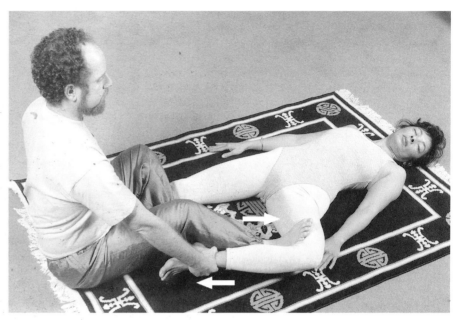

Fig. 19A

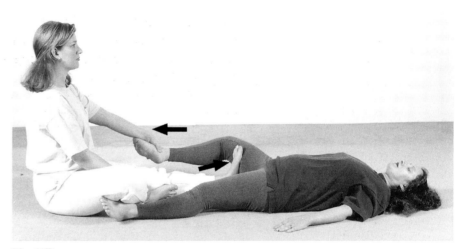

Fig. 19B

19. Sit between the client's legs, take hold of the ankle of the bent leg and place your other hand near the ankle of the straight leg. Foot press into the medial thigh of the client, starting in the area behind the knee, moving halfway up the thigh and then back toward the knee. With each press of the foot, lean back and simultaneously pull at the ankle of the bent leg in order to deepen the stretch. Repeat.

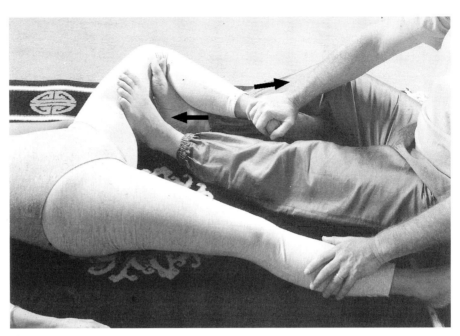

Fig. 20

20. Place the foot of the client's bent leg under your knee and clasp the foot at the ankle. Use your other foot to foot press into the thigh, starting halfway up and continuing to just distal to the groin area, in positions 1, 2, 3, 2, 1. With each press in with the foot, pull at the ankle of the bent leg, creating a counter-force, in order to deepen the stretch.

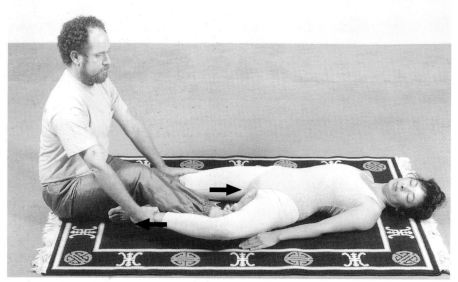

Fig. 21A

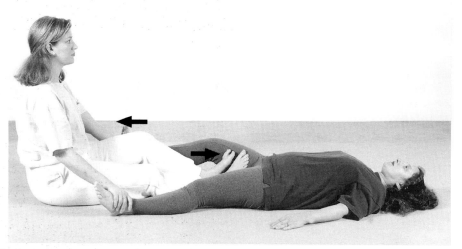

Fig. 21B

21. Remove the bent leg from behind your knee and continue holding at the ankle. Press with both feet in an alternating pattern into the medial thigh of the bent leg while simultaneously pulling at the ankle of the bent leg. Repeat as many times as desired.

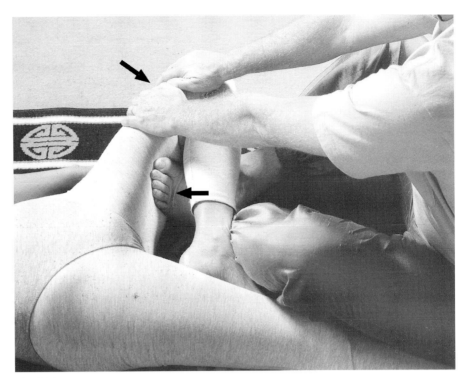

Fig. 22A

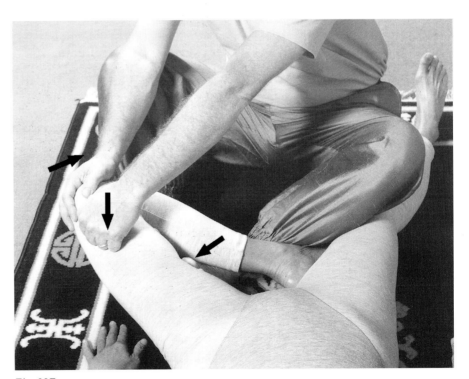

Fig. 22B

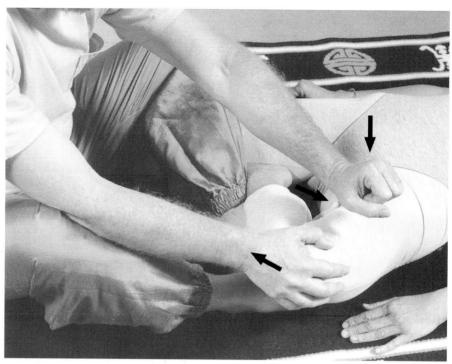

Fig. 22C

22. Release the ankle and slide forward, keeping your feet against the client's thigh. The client's leg is bent and is held in place by your knee. Lean back, pushing into the thigh with your feet while simultaneously pulling with your hands across the thigh of the bent leg. Work with the hands together on the thigh and then with the hands in an alternating pattern. Make a loose fist and percuss the lateral surface of the thigh of the bent leg.

23. Kneel and place the upright bent leg of the client securely between your thighs. Work with a press and pull with the fingertips of both hands on the medial and lateral number 1 Sen lines of the leg from the knee to the hip.

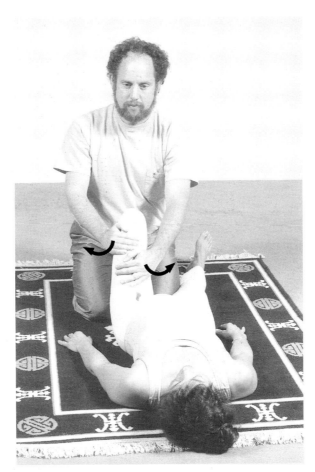

Fig. 23A

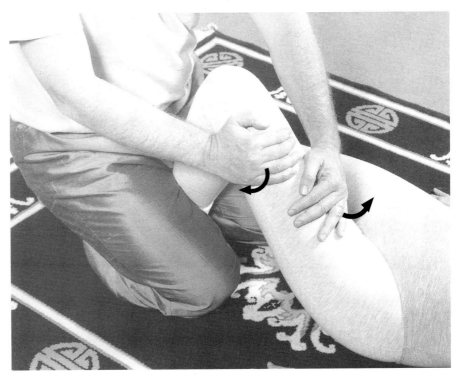

Fig. 23B

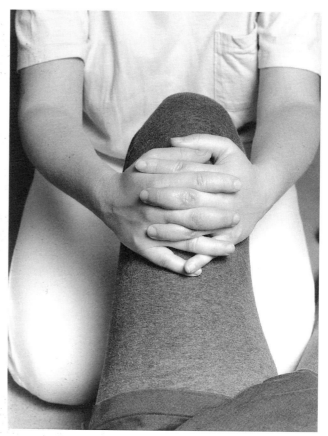

Fig. 24A

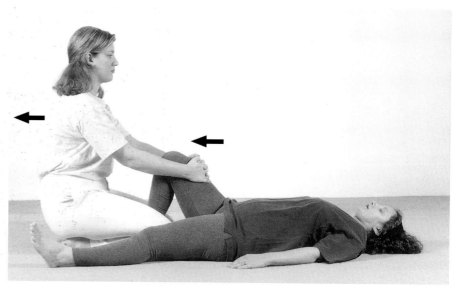

Fig. 24B

24. Interlace your fingers and use the heels of the hands to work Sen line number 2 on both the medial and lateral thigh.

Squeeze in with the heels of the hands and lean back, pulling the client's body slightly up, providing a stretch into the low back.

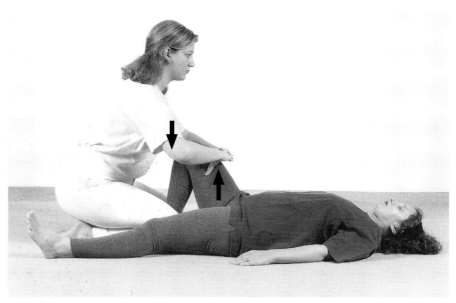

Fig. 25A

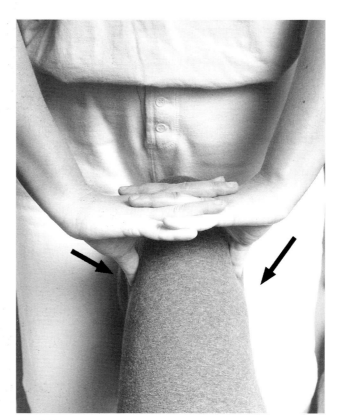

Fig. 25B

25. Keep your fingers interlocked. Rotate the hands so that the thumbs point down. Thumb press into lines 3 on both the inside and outside of the thigh. (The pressure is achieved by slowly lowering the elbows, not by direct pressure with the thumbs alone.) Work from the knee proximally and then return distally to the knee region.

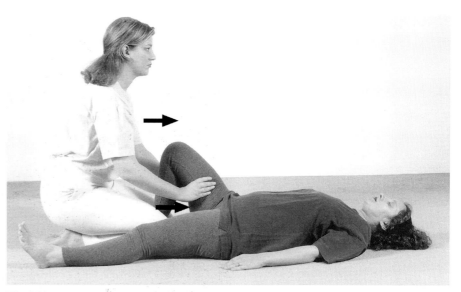

Fig. 26A

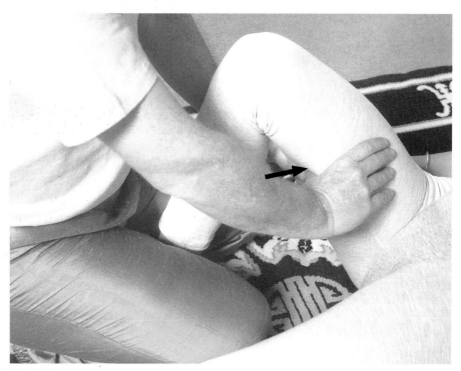

Fig. 26B

26. Move the client's foot slightly forward thereby opening up the region of the posterior thigh. Placing one thumb over the other thumb, thumb press down the center line of the posterior thigh to the hamstring muscle attachments and then back up to the area behind the knee. With each thumb press, lean forward to press deeply into this big muscle group.

Repeat working down and up this center line, now using the thumb-chasing-thumb technique. This will be with less pressure than the thumb-on-thumb technique.

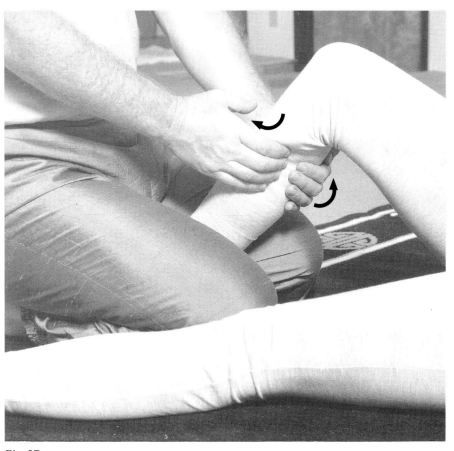

Fig. 27

27. Use your fingertips to divide the gastrocnemius muscle. Alternate hands, pulling to the left and then to the right, leaning back with each pull of the muscle. Work from the knee distally and then back proximally. Place the palm of one hand over the back of the other hand and palm press the gastrocnemius, pushing the muscle into the bones of the lower leg.

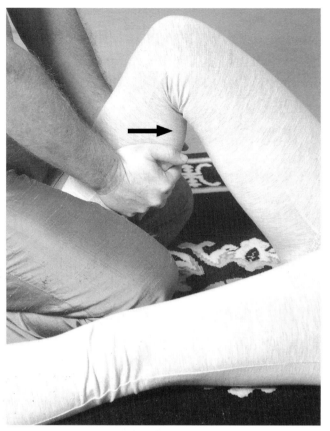

Fig. 28

28. Interlock your fingers, grab the gastrocnemius with the heels of the hands, squeeze and lean forward, pulling the muscle away from the bone.

Repeat the procedure moving distally and then proximally.

Release the fingers and utilize gentle palm circles along both sides of the gastrocnemius for relaxation.

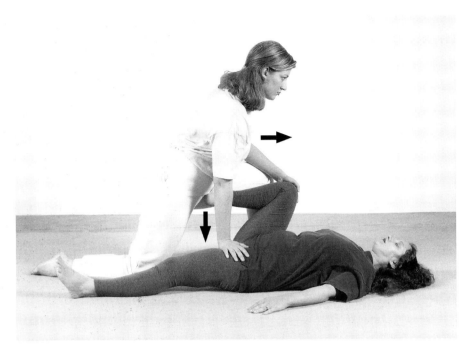

Fig. 29

29. Take up a kneeling position, with one leg at a 90° angle, the foot flat on the futon. Place the client's foot into the inguinal region of the side of the leg that is at 90°. Place one hand over the knee of the client's bent leg, and the other hand proximal to the knee of the straight leg. Shift your weight forward, bringing the client's knee toward the chest while simultaneously palm pressing straight down into the thigh of the straight leg.

Repeat this procedure in a pattern of palm presses in positions 1, 2, 3, 2, 1 on the straight leg. With each shift forward, attempt to move the client's knee closer to his or her chest.

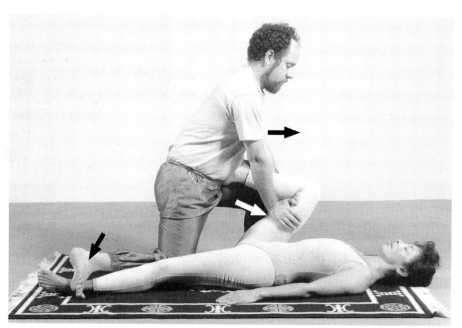

Fig. 30

30. Move the foot of your bent leg out slightly to the side and place both palms together on the posterior thigh of the client's bent leg. Palm press on the back of the thigh from the area behind the knee to the ischial tuberosity and back to the knee in the pattern 1, 2, 3, 2, 1. (Note the practitioner holding the client's straight leg in place by placing his ankle across the client's ankle.)

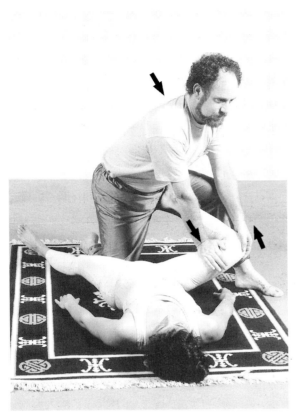

Fig. 31A

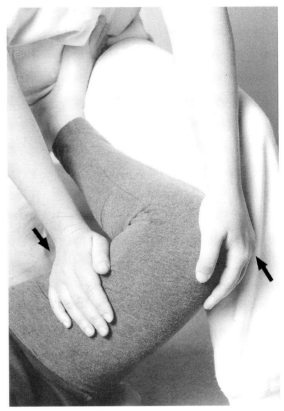

Fig. 31B

31. Move the foot of your bent leg laterally while retaining the client's foot in your inguinal area. This allows the client to open up their pelvic region. Hold the knee of the client's bent leg securely with your hand. With your other hand, palm press the medial thigh of the bent leg, working in the pattern 1, 2, 3, 2, 1. Depending on the flexibility of the client, his or her knee can potentially reach all the way to the futon. With each palm press, lift up at the knee, providing a counter-force and a deepening of the compression.

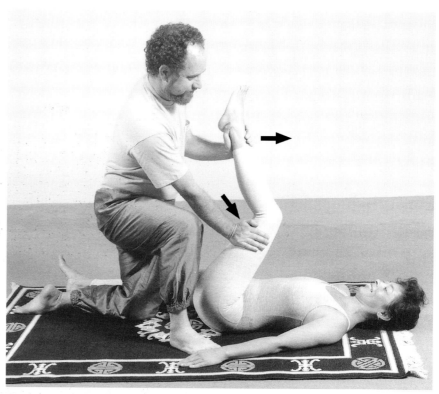

Fig. 32

32. Straighten the client's leg and hold at the ankle. Palm press into the hamstring muscle. While retaining the deep palm press, push the client's ankle forward and slightly across the body, aiming toward the eye on the opposite side of his or her body.

Palm press from the area posterior to the knee proximal to the ischial tuberosity and back in the pattern 1, 2, 3, 2, 1. While holding each palm press, the ankle is brought forward toward the head.

Upon completion of the palm presses, continue holding the leg at the ankle and make a loose fist with your other hand; percuss the entire length of the client's leg.

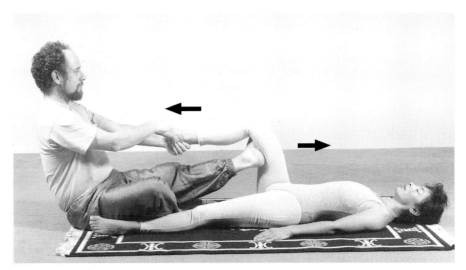

Fig. 33A

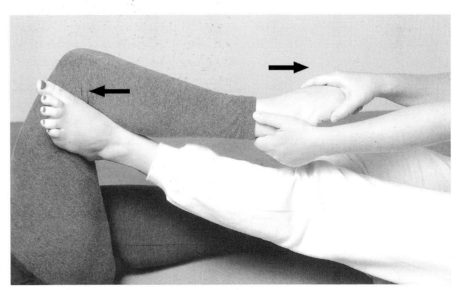

Fig. 33B

33. Sit and hold the client's leg at a 90° angle. Place your foot just proximal to the knee of the client's bent leg with the toes pointed outward. Press into the posterior thigh with your foot while simultaneously pulling at the ankle. The stretch is enhanced by extending the client's toes downward at the conclusion of the pull on the ankle. The foot presses in three positions, from just proximal to the knee to halfway down the thigh.

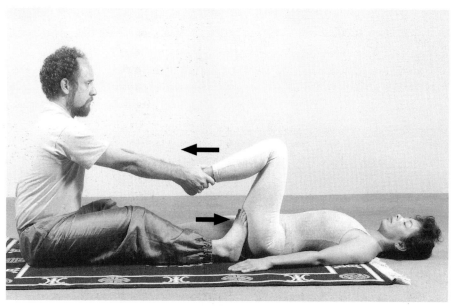

Fig. 34

34. Place your foot flat against the client's posterior thigh with your heel on the futon. Press in with the entire foot while simultaneously pulling at the ankle, extending the toes downward and leaning back.

Next, come forward and push the client's knee towards his or her chest while keeping the foot in the same position. The foot position automatically lowers as the thigh is repositioned against the foot.

The procedure is repeated with the foot in the second position: pressing in with foot, pulling at the ankle, and extending the client's toes downward.

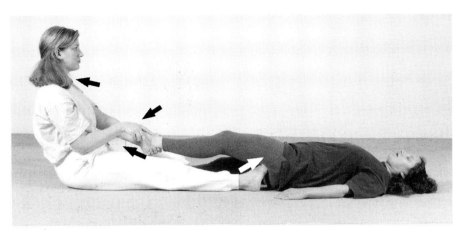

Fig. 35A

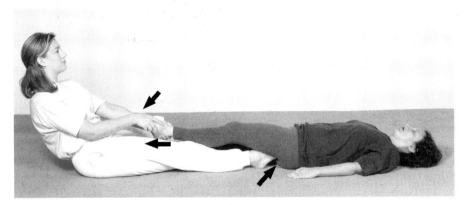

Fig. 35B

35. Again, push the client's knee toward his or her chest, changing the relative position of the foot into a third position with the toes against the ischial tuberosity.

Repeat the procedures a third time, pressing in with the foot as you lean back, pulling at the ankle and extending the toes.

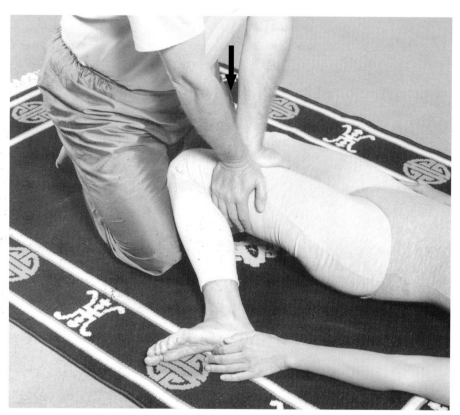

Fig. 36

36. In a kneeling position, take the bent leg of the client and position the leg so that the heel is in the vicinity of the client's own buttocks. You can use your own knees to support the client's knee if he or she is not able to stretch comfortably into this position. Palm press with one hand from the foot of the bent leg to the knee, and with the other hand palm press the thigh from the inguinal area to the knee.

Bring both hands together and palm press on the thigh from the knee up to the inguinal area, working in positions 1, 2, 3, 2 1.

Bring the palms of your hands together and percuss along the thigh. Holding at the ankle and the knee, straighten the client's leg.

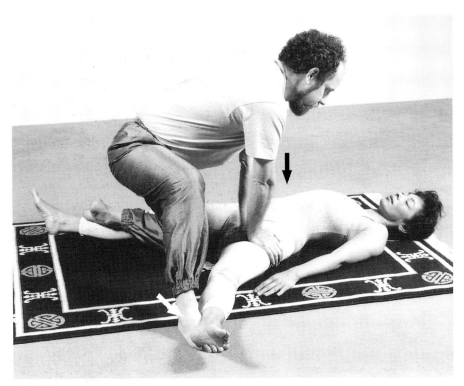

Fig. 37A

37. Extend the client's leg laterally three times and at the maximum stretch place your ankle against the ankle of the client, fixing the leg in place. Palm press with both hands the thigh of the extended leg in positions 1, 2, 3, 2, 1.

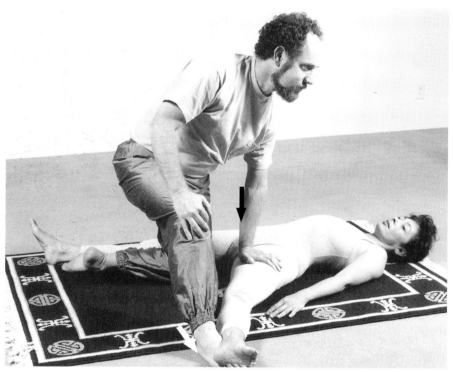

Fig. 37B

Continue with palm presses with one hand up to the pulse point in the inguinal area. At the place where the pulse of the femoral artery can be palpated (the end point of Sen line 2), press down deeply with the heel of the hand, obstructing the pulse for up to 10 seconds. Release slowly and palm press back down to just proximal to the knee. (***The stopping of the blood flow is contraindicated with clients with heart problems and circulation problems into the legs.***)

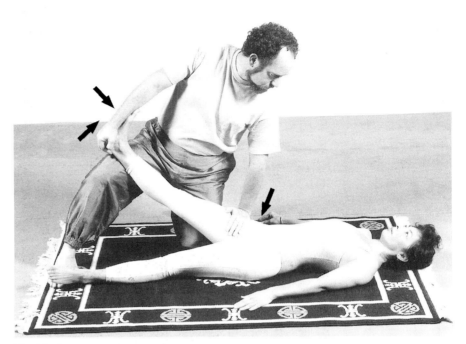

Fig. 38

38. Move laterally to a position outside the client's legs. Hold the heel of the client's foot in the palm of your hand with the toes against your forearm. Place the other hand distal to the inguinal area of the same leg. Simultaneously, palm press from the inguinal area to just above the knee in positions 1, 2, 3, 2, 1 while also doing an Achilles tendon stretch by lifting the heel and pressing the forearm into the toes. With each palm press and Achilles tendon stretch, lean laterally in the direction of the client's head.

Change legs and repeat procedures 17 through 38.

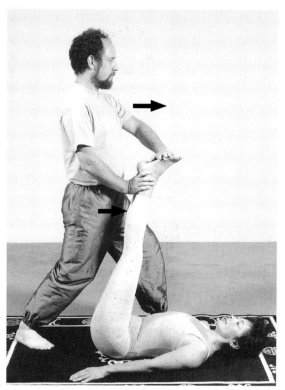

Fig. 39A

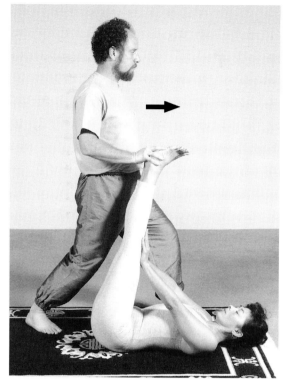

Fig. 39B

39. Stand and assume a bow stance with your outside leg forward, the foot near the client's shoulder. Bring the client's legs to a 90° angle to the futon. Holding at the ankles, shift your weight forward, bringing the client's feet in the direction of the head.

Repeat three times, the third time extending the feet closest to the client's head. The client's hands can be placed on the knees, elbows straight. This creates a counter-force to the practitioner's action and increases the stretch. To increase the stretch even more, the client can place his or her hands on the thighs as the practitioner brings the feet forward.

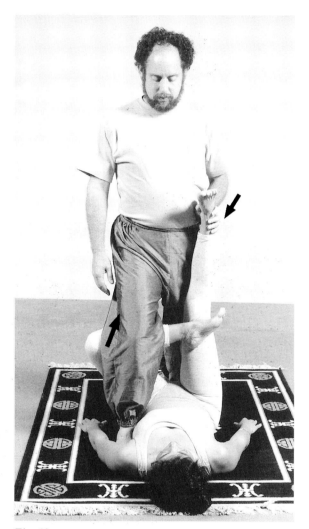

Fig. 40

40. The client is in a modified half-lotus position, with one leg held straight up at 90° to the futon and the other leg bent, and with the ankle of the bent leg positioned in the vicinity of the knee of the straight leg. Step forward, placing your leg over the client's bent leg. Hold at the ankle of the vertical leg and push the leg forward three times, with the third time being the strongest. The client's bent leg is held in position by your leg.

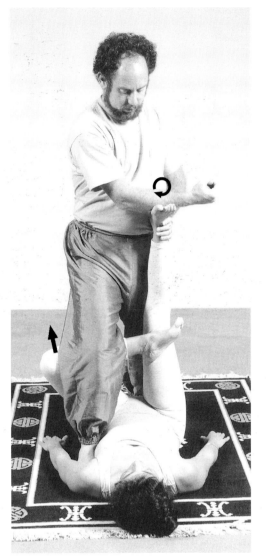
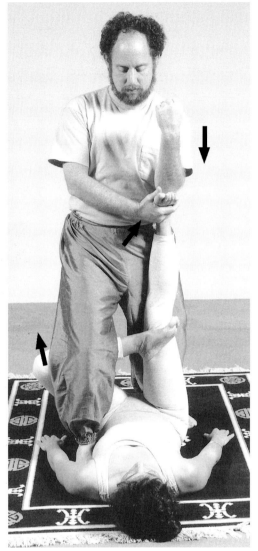

Fig. 41A   *Fig. 41B*

41. Step forward with your back leg in order to support the client's vertical leg. Roll the bottom of the foot with your forearm while supporting the top of the foot with your other hand.

Press down into the bottom of the foot with your elbow into six points (see procedure 4, page 38, for the locations of the six points). Hold the elbow press for 5 seconds and release by bringing the hand forward.

42. After all six points have been treated with the elbow, roll the bottom of the foot with the forearm for integration.

Step back, bringing your leg away from the client's bent leg. Make a loose fist and percuss the bottom of the foot and then the entire straight leg.

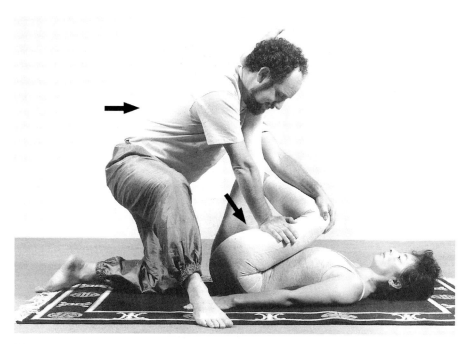

Fig. 43

43. Step back and kneel down onto one knee. The client's leg is vertical and rests against your shoulder. Hold the knee of the client's bent leg with the hand on the same side as where the straight leg is resting. Your other hand is placed on the posterior thigh of the bent leg just below the knee. Shift your weight forward, bringing the straight leg toward the client's head, while simultaneously palm pressing on the posterior thigh, working in a pattern 1, 2, 3, 2, 1. The vector of each palm press is on a slight angle aimed at the sternum of the client.

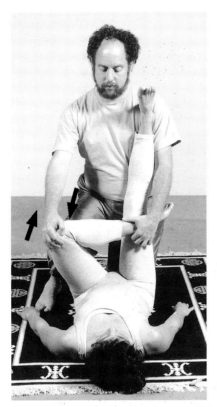

Fig. 44A

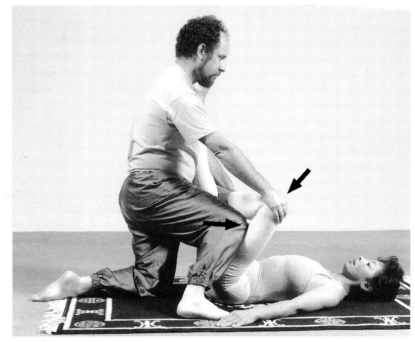

Fig. 44B

44. Place the hand you were using to palm press in 43, above, on the knee of the client's bent leg. Your other hand holds the ankle of the bent leg. Place the knee of the leg that is at 90° into the posterior thigh of the client's bent leg just below the knee. Simultaneously, push into the posterior thigh with your knee and pull back at the client's knee with your hand.

Repeat this in positions 1, 2, 3, 2, 1 on the posterior thigh.

Change legs and repeat procedures 40 through 44 on the other side.

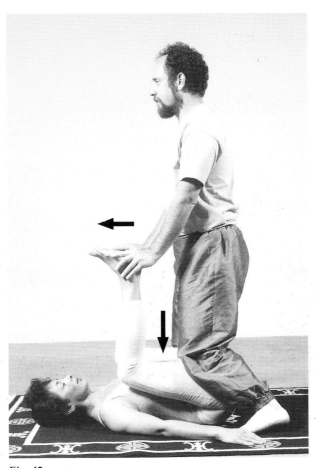

Fig. 45

Procedures 45 and 46 are prohibited during pregnancy.

45. Stand and hold both of the client's legs at the ankles. Bend your legs, placing your knees into the attachments of the hamstring muscles at the ischial tuberosities. Let your weight sink down into the hamstrings and then bring the client's feet forward in the direction of his or her head.

Lift your knees up slightly and reposition them in position 2, distal to the hamstring attachments. Sink your weight down into the muscle and then push the client's feet forward.

Lift the knees, reposition them on the midpoint of the hamstring muscles at position 3, sink down and bring the feet forward.

Repeat the procedures again at position 2, and finish at position 1, at the hamstring attachments.

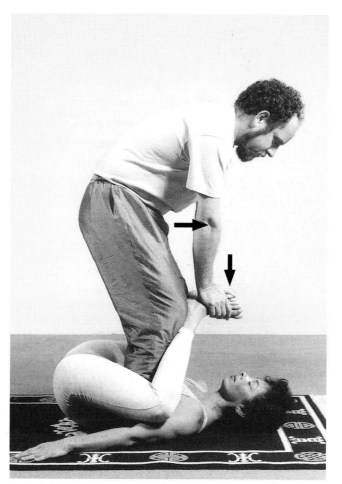

Fig. 46A

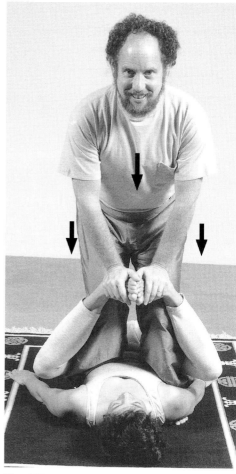

Fig. 46B

46. Hold the client's legs at the ankles, step forward between the client's legs, and place your feet under the axillary region of the client. Bring the soles of the client's feet together just in front of your abdomen.

Bend your knees, sinking downward and simultaneously push the feet of the client forward and down in the direction of his or her head. This lifts the client's hips off the futon.

Repeat the procedure three times.

Step back, placing your toes where your heels were previously.

Repeat three times with the feet in the new position.

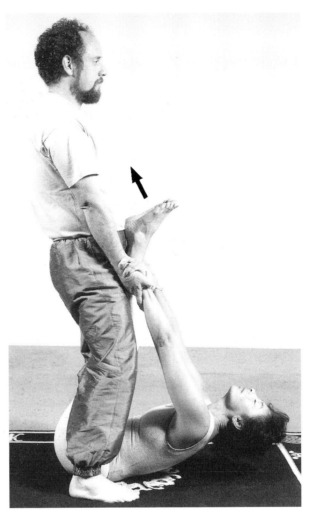

Fig. 47

47. Stand with your feet on either side of the client's hips. The client's legs are held vertically, resting against your abdomen. Practitioner and client hold each other's forearms by wrapping their fingers around the other person's forearms just proximal to the wrists. Lean back and pull the client's upper body forward and up. Repeat three times.

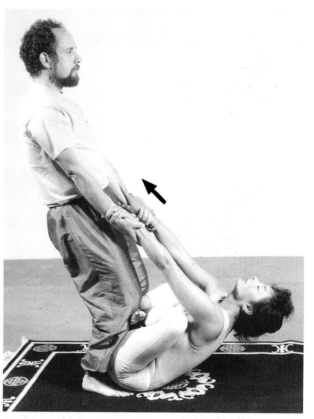

Fig. 48

48. The client crosses his or her legs into a half or full lotus position. Place your lower legs against the crossed legs of the client. Once again, practitioner and client hold each other's forearms. Lean back and pull the client up. Repeat twice.

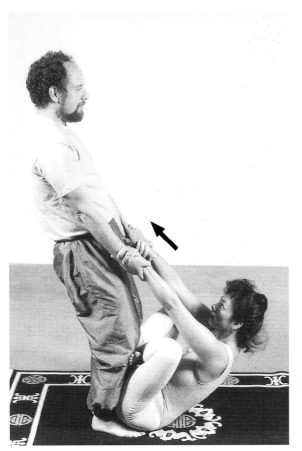

Fig. 49A

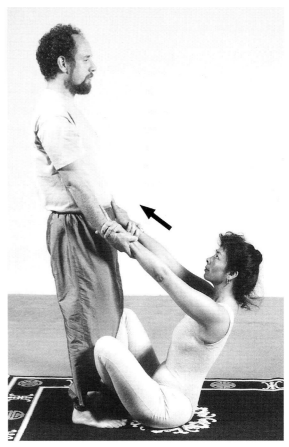

Fig. 49B

49. Procedure 49 is a continuation of procedure 48 above. Pull the client up a third time and step back a few steps, bringing the client into a seated position.

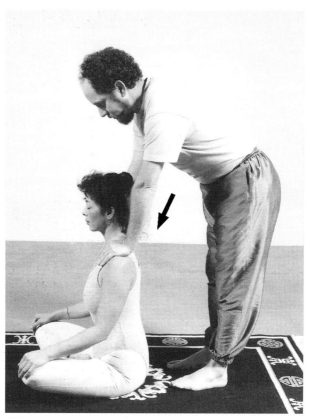

Fig. 50

50. Stand behind the seated client. Starting on either side of the neck, palm press into both shoulders simultaneously, moving laterally to the acromial extremities and back toward the neck in positions 1, 2, 3, 2, 1. The client places his or her hands in front of the body to provide a counter-force. Palm press down and up the back on either side of the spine. Place your palms together and percuss the entire back and shoulder region with a chopping motion. Utilizing the hands separately, gently brush the back from the shoulders to the hips.

The abdominal region

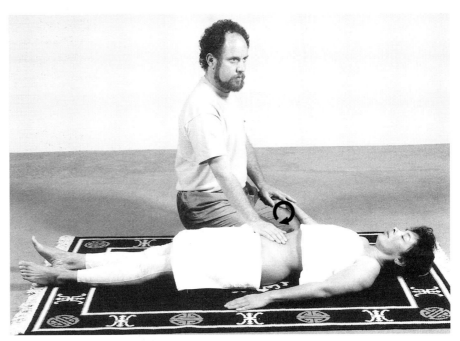

Fig. 51A

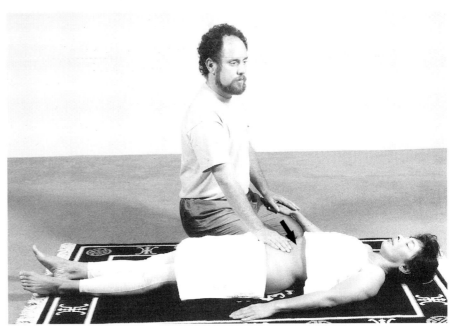

Fig. 51B

51. The abdominal region is defined superiorly by the lower border of the ribcage; laterally by the mid-axillary line; and inferiorally by the pubic bone.

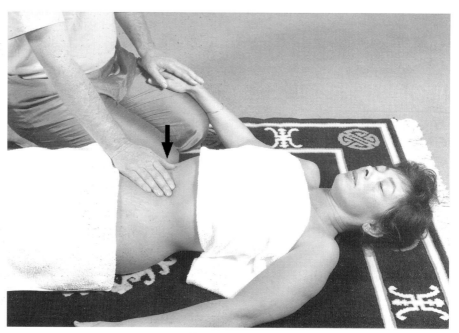

Fig. 51C

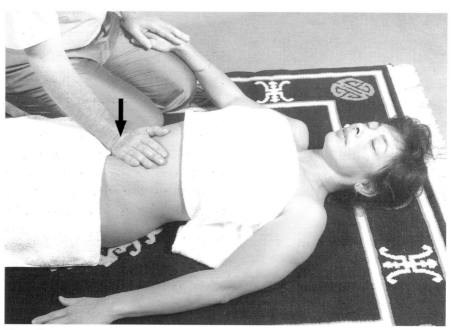

Fig. 51D

The client lies in a supine position, preferably with knees raised by a pillow. Kneel at the client's right side. Make small clockwise palm circles, moving in a general clockwise direction, beginning on the midline below the navel, working up the right side of the client's abdomen, across just below the ribcage, and continuing down the client's left side. The palm circles can be repeated many times with the intention of relaxing the abdominal muscles and increasing the blood and lymph flow in the region.

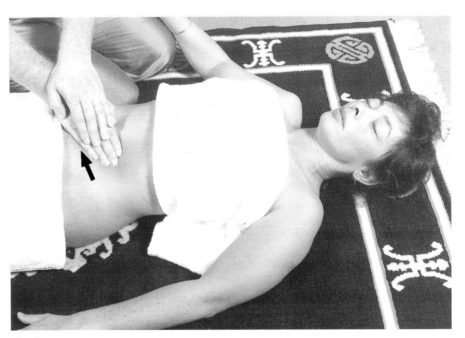

Fig. 51E

Visualize the abdominal region divided into nine equal zones with the navel being in the center. Zone 1 is below the navel on the client's right side, just medial to the anterior superior iliac spine.

In each of the nine zones, deep press with the heel of the hand directed toward the navel, while the client makes an exhalation. Hold each deep press for up to 30 seconds, depending on the client's comfort level. At the end of the 30 seconds, instruct the client to take a big inhalation into the abdomen. As the breath fills the abdomen, slowly allow your hand to come up. With the subsequent exhalation, reach across the navel with your fingertips, compress slightly, and drag your fingertips back toward the navel.

Repeat for zones 2 through 9.

Upon completion of the deep palm presses in the nine zones, do gentle palm circles clockwise around the entire abdominal region.

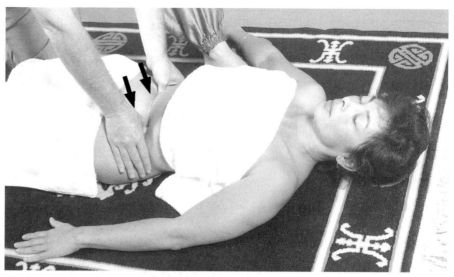

Fig. 52

52. Identify six points in the vicinity of the client's navel. Using the length of the client's thumb as a measuring tool, measure from the center of the navel laterally to both sides to determine the first two points (3 and 4). Superior to the navel, two points (1 and 2) are determined using the length of the client's thumb measuring superior to the first two points that were located lateral to the navel. Points 5 and 6 are located a thumb length lateral and a thumb length inferior to the navel.

Beginning with points 1 and 2, ask the client to exhale. With the exhalation, sink deeply with thumb presses into points 1 and 2. Hold for up to 30 seconds. Complete the procedure by asking the client to take a big inhalation while you slowly remove your thumbs from the deep compression.

Repeat the procedure at points 3 and 4 just lateral to the navel, and finally at points 5 and 6, inferior and lateral to the navel.

After completion of the deep thumb presses, integrate the work with gentle palm circles around the entire abdominal region.

Finally place the palm of your left hand directly over the navel and your right palm over the back of your left hand. With an exhalation, palm press down with moderate pressure to create a centering and a quieting sensation. Retain the press for up to 30 seconds and release with a big inhalation by the client.

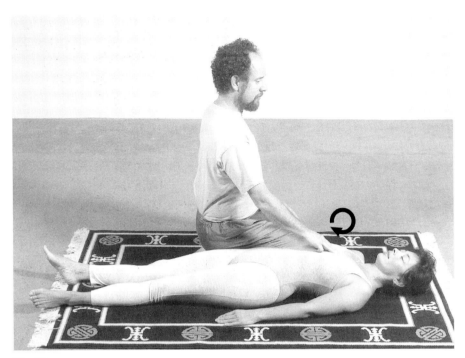

Fig. 53

53. Use the three middle fingers of one hand to make finger circles in a clockwise rotation from the xiphoid process up the sternum to the sternoclavicular notch. The finger circles are continued back down the sternum and then back up.

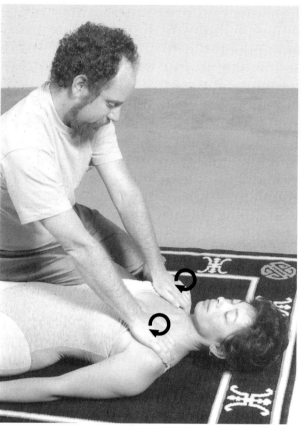

Fig. 54

54. Make finger circles with both hands from the midline, working laterally along the lower border of the clavicle. Continue with finger circles medially and laterally in the intercostal space below the clavicle.

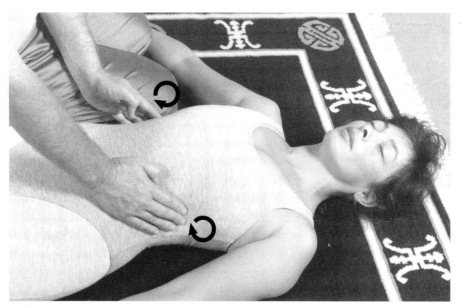

Fig. 55

55. Make finger circles or thumb circles in the intercostal spaces of the entire ribcage, working laterally from the sternum to the mid-axillary line and then back medially to the edge of the sternum.

Make palm circles along the mid-axillary line on both sides of the client.

Chest, shoulders, neck and arms

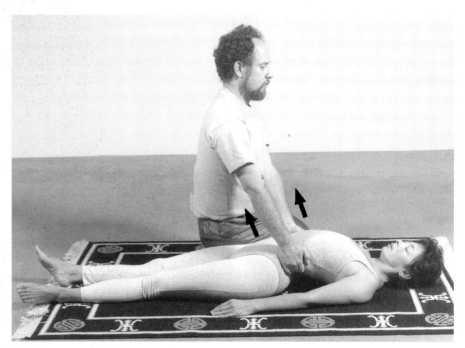

Fig. 56

56. Reach under the client on both sides, just below the ribs. Lean back and lift with both hands, bringing the client's mid-section up off the futon.

Repeat the lean and lift in two other locations; the most distal location is just above the crest of the pelvis and the middle location is halfway between the bottom of the ribs and the pelvis.

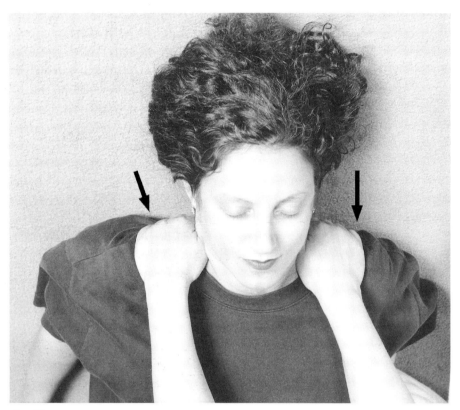

Fig. 57

57. Make finger circles with three fingers, working up the sternum to the sternoclavicular notch; then utilize both hands to do finger circles laterally to the shoulders.

At the shoulders, palm press into the pectoralis muscles and over the shoulder joint.

Hook your fingers under the upper trapezius muscles and lean back, stretching the shoulders and neck. Repeat the hook and lean three times, moving from the nape of the neck laterally toward the acromial extremity.

Palm press the shoulders and upper chest region for integration.

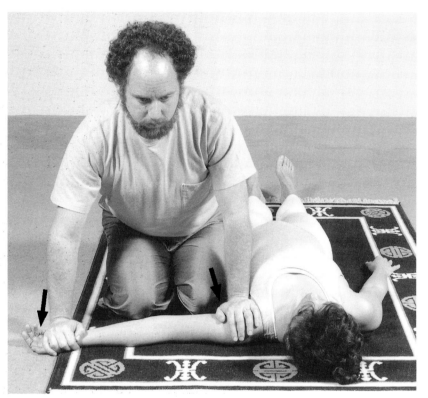

Fig. 58

58. The client's arm is extended out to the side, with the palmar surface facing up. Place one hand at the wrist and the other hand in the axillary region. Leaning forward, push in at the axilla and extend outward at the wrist, creating a stretch and elongation of the client's arm. Repeat the stretch three times.

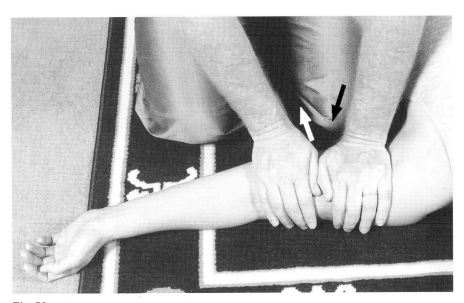

Fig. 59

59. Palm press from the axillary region to the elbow with one hand and from the palm to the elbow with the other hand. The hands come together near the elbow and you then palm press the entire arm distally, then proximally, and again distally, finishing at the wrist.

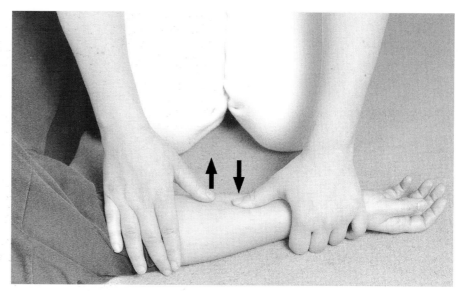

Fig. 60

60. Thumb press in the pattern of thumb-chasing-thumb, from the wrist joint between the tendons palmaris longus and flexor carpi radials, to the elbow.

Above the elbow, thumb press up to the axillary region, working either above the humerus bone or just below the bone in the sulcus of the muscle.

Thumb press back down the arm to the wrist, utilizing the thumb-chasing-thumb pattern.

Integrate the thumb presses with palm presses, working proximal to the axillary region.

 In the axillary region, locate the axillary artery and utilizing the heel of the hand, press in, obstructing the artery for 10–30 seconds. Release slowly from the artery and then palm press back down the arm. *Stopping the blood flow at the axillary is contraindicated with any heart problems.*

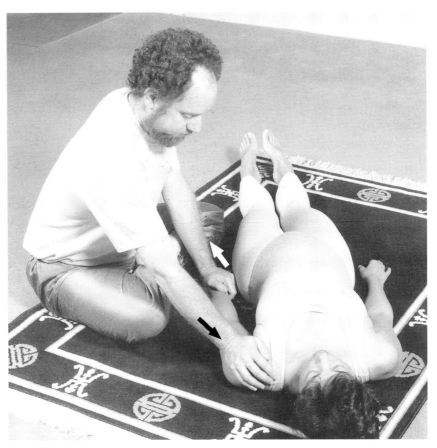

Fig. 61

61. Position the client's arm along his or her side, parallel to the body, with the palmar surface down. Place one of your hands at the wrist and the other at the shoulder. Pulling at the wrist and holding at the shoulder, stretch the client's arm.

With one hand, palm press from the shoulder to elbow, and with the other hand from the wrist to the elbow. The hands come together at the elbow; you then palm press the entire arm, finishing at the wrist.

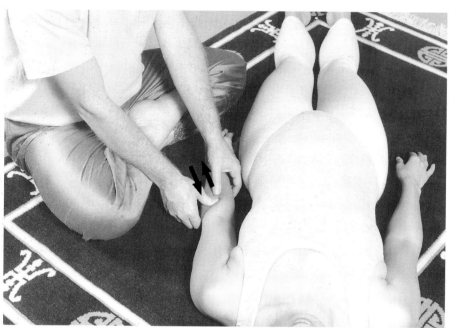

Fig. 62

62. Starting just proximal to the wrist, between the radius and ulna, use the thumb-chasing-thumb technique up the midline of the forearm to the elbow. Above the elbow, thumb press either above or below the humerus up to the acromial extremity. Use the thumb-chases-thumb technique again back down the arm, and then integrate the procedure with palm presses up and back down the arm to the wrist.

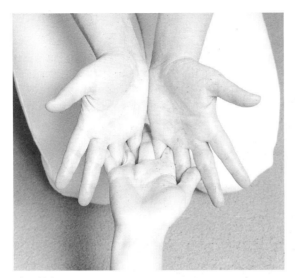

Fig. 63A

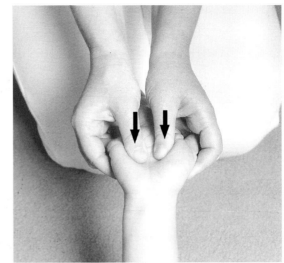

Fig. 63B

63. Palm press the palmar surface of the client's hand.

Using both hands, interlock your fingers with the fingers of the client's hand. Thumb press deeply into six points on the palmar surface of the client's hand. Thumb press all around the palm of the client's hand.

Use the heels of your hands to firmly rub and press into the client's palm.

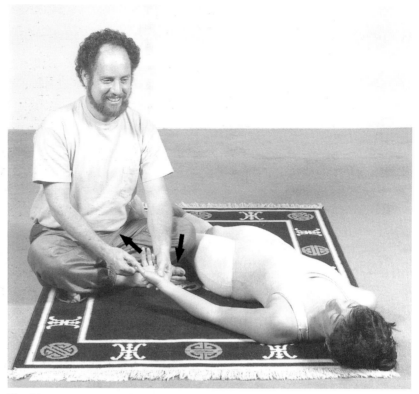

Fig. 64

64. With one hand, hold the client's hand at the wrist, palmar surface up. Thumb press at the point (acupoint Pericardium 7 Daling) on the wrist crease between the tendons palmaris longus and flexor digitorum longus. Continue with thumb presses into the palm and then switch to finger circles when you reach the phalange bones of the thumb.

Finger circle along the thumb and finish by pressing the tip of the thumb.

Repeat the procedures, one finger at a time, for the other four fingers: thumb press at the wrist, thumb press in the palm, finger circle out each finger, and press at the finger tip.

Finally, palm press the entire palm for integration of the work.

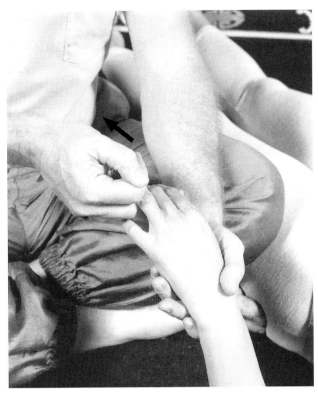

Fig. 65

65. Rotate the client's hand so that the back of the hand faces up. Thumb press into the point on the midline of the wrist crease. Make thumb circles along the back of the hand and onto the thumb. Upon reaching the end of the thumb, grasp the thumb and pull.

Repeat the procedures for the other fingers: press at the wrist, finger circles on the back of the hand and along each finger individually, followed by a pull on the finger. When treating the little finger, make the finger circles along the outside of the hand along the little finger.

Palm press on the back of the hand for integration of the detailed work.

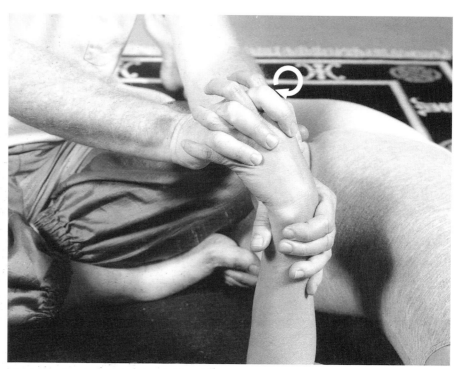

Fig. 66

66. Hold the hand at the wrist with one hand and interlace fingers with the client with the other hand. Rotate the client's wrist five times clockwise and five times counter-clockwise. Remove the interlaced fingers by very slowly dragging them apart.

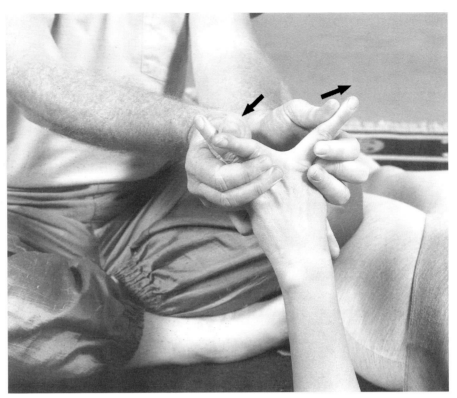

Fig. 67

67. Slowly stretch the client's fingers apart two at a time.

Work on each finger individually, putting the finger between your own index and middle finger, making circles and pulling. At the distal aspect of the finger, quickly slide off the finger, creating a snapping sensation.

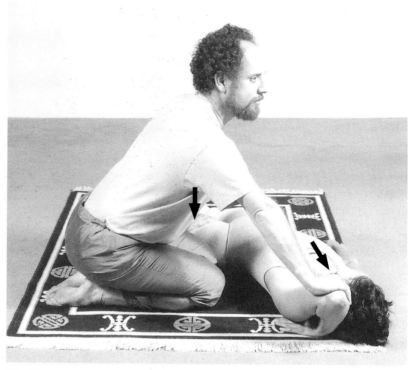

Fig. 68

68. Lift the arm, placing the palm downward next to the side of the head, the fingers pointing back toward the feet, and with the elbow pointing upward. Place one hand on the upper arm proximal to the elbow and your other hand on the upper thigh on the same side.

Press the elbow downward toward the top of the head while simultaneously palm pressing on the thigh in positions 1, 2, 3, 2, 1 from the upper thigh to just superior to the knee and back, creating an elongation along the mid-axillary line of the body.

Hold the elbow with one hand and massage the triceps muscle of the bent arm with the other hand.

Lift and straighten the bent arm, gently shake it, and place the arm along the client's side.

Repeat procedures 58 through 68 on the other arm.

Face and neck

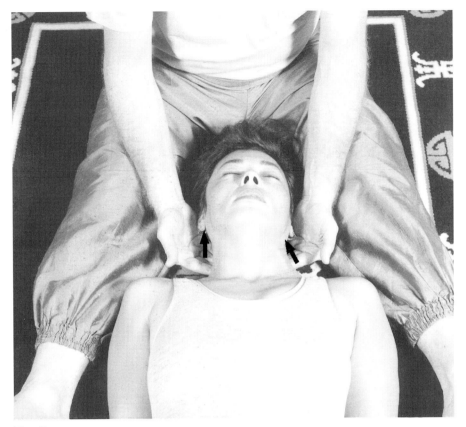

Fig. 69

69. Kneel or sit at the client's head. Palm press both shoulders, pressing down in the direction of the feet, from the nape of the neck laterally to the acromial extremity and then back to the neck.

Thumb press into the muscles of both shoulders, working laterally to the acromial extremity and then back medially to the neck. Palm press the shoulders for integration of the detailed pressing.

Reach under the neck from both sides with the fingers, pressing and pulling up along the trapezius and levator scapulae muscles, creating an extension and elongation of the neck. Starting on the midline, just below the occipital protuberance, press with the fingertips along the occipital ridge working laterally to the mastoid processes. With the pressing, also lift the head slightly to enhance the extension.

Hold the head in one hand and turn it slightly to the side. With the other hand, make finger circles down the sternocleidomastoid (SCM) muscle of the neck.

Switch hands, turn the head in the other direction, and make finger circles down the SCM on the second side.

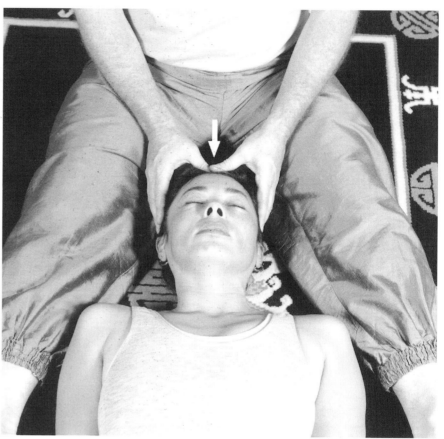

Fig. 70A

70. Press with your fingertips from the hollow just below the occipital protuberance up the back of the head to the crown of the head, then back down to the hollow; repeat the presses back to the crown.

At the crown, switch to the thumb-on-thumb technique and press from the crown to the hairline on the midline of the head and back to the crown.

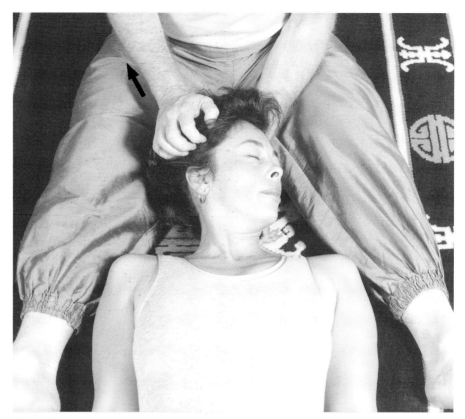

Fig. 70B

Hold the head in one hand and utilizes the other hand to make finger circles through the scalp. Scratch the scalp and gently pull the hair from the roots.

Switch hands to finger circle and scratch the scalp, and pull the hair on the second side of the head. Finger circle across the forehead and on the templar region.

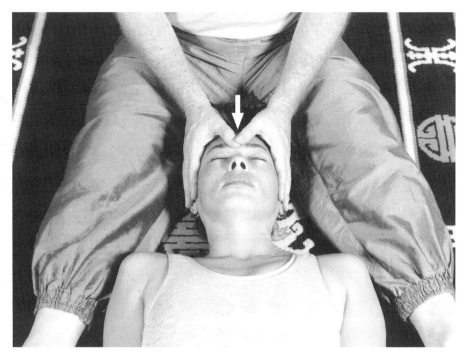

Fig. 71A

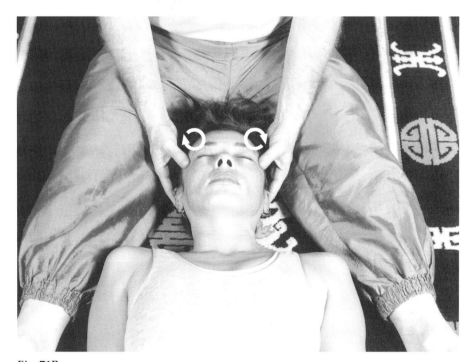

Fig. 71B

71. Thumb press along both eyebrows to the temples. At the temples, make thumb or finger circles.

Thumb press along the orbit bones of the eyes, the zygomatic arches, and along the nose.

At the termination of presses on each aspect of the face, make slow circles in the temple region for integration.

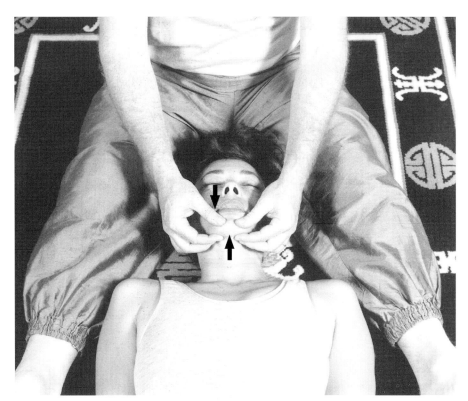

Fig. 72

72. To treat the masseter muscles of the jaw and the chin, squeeze the muscle tissue between your thumbs and fingers to create a pinching sensation. Return to the temple area and make thumb or finger circles for integration.

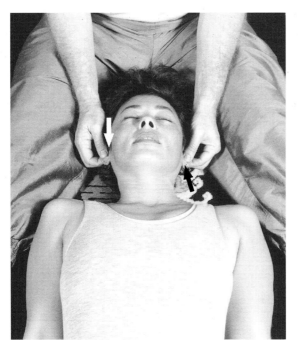

Fig. 73A

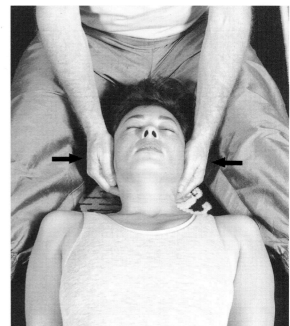

Fig. 73B

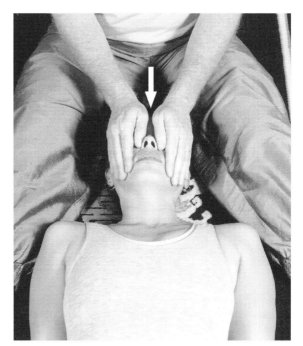

Fig. 73C

73. Massage the external auricles of the ears. Cup the palms of your hands over the client's ears, obstructing the hearing and hold for up to 30 seconds. Remove the hands and repeat covering the ears twice more.

Palm press the shoulders.

Lift the head with both hands, lean back, pulling the head, and traction the neck. Complete the head and neck work with gentle palm presses on the shoulders. Rub together the palms of your hands, creating a gentle heat from the friction. Gently place the palms of your hands over the client's eyes and remain in this position for 20–30 seconds.

4 Client in lateral recumbent position

Legs

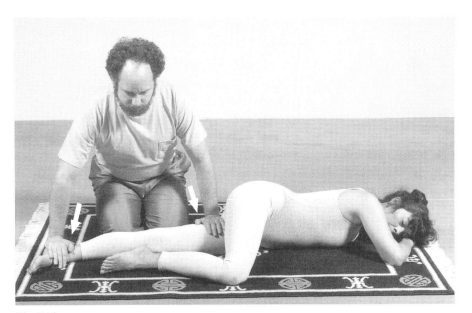

Fig. 74A

74. The client lies on his or her side in a lateral recumbent position, with the bottom leg straight and the upper leg bent. Palm press on both legs from the ankles up to the hips and then back to the ankles.

Kneel or sit behind the client, holding the ankle with one hand and at the muscle attachments at the gluteal fold with the other hand, and stretch the straight leg. Palm press from the ankle to the knee with one hand and from the hip to the knee with the other hand.

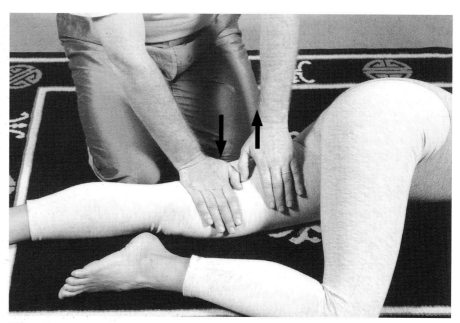

Fig. 74B

At the knee, palm press up and down the entire straight leg with the hands together.

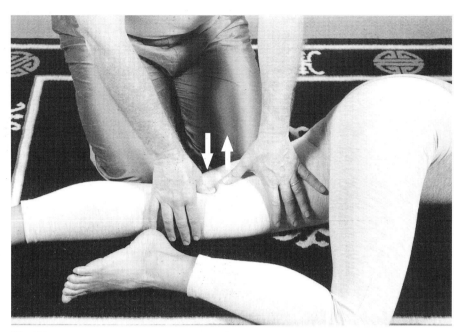

Fig. 75

75. Thumb press, utilizing the thumb-chasing-thumb pattern, up and down the three Sen lines on the medial surface of the straight leg (see page 47).

Palm press up the straight leg and at the end of Sen line 2, hold a deep palm press for 10 seconds, slowly release, and palm press down the leg. *The deep palm press is contraindicated with clients having high blood pressure or heart problems.*

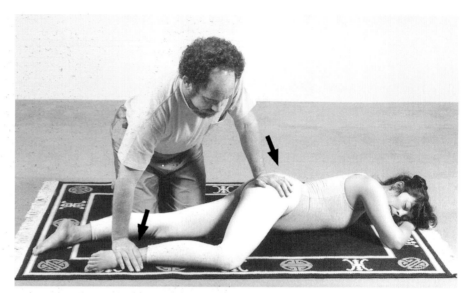

Fig. 76A

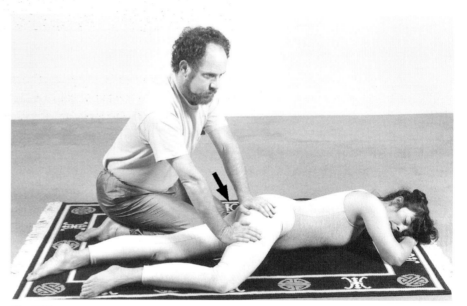

Fig. 76B

76. Reach across the client's straight leg and hold the ankle of the bent leg with one hand; place the other hand on the client's hip. Pull at the ankle while stabilizing the leg at the hip, creating an extension of the client's leg.

Palm press from the ankle to the knee with one hand and from the hip to the knee with the other hand. The hands come together at the knee and you then palm press up and back down the bent leg.

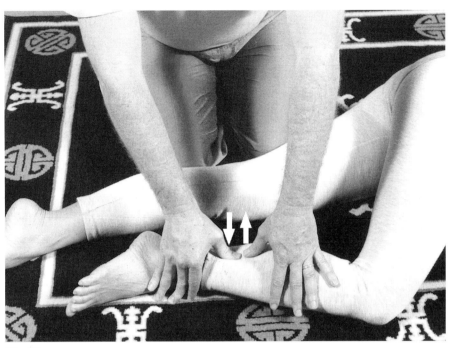

Fig. 77

77. Thumb press utilizing the thumb-chasing-thumb technique up and down the lateral aspect of the bent leg on Sen lines 2 and 3 (see pages 47–48). Palm press up and down the bent leg for integration.

Stretches applied with the feet

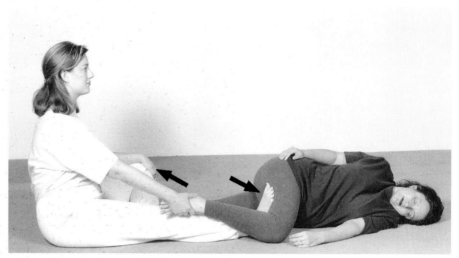

Fig. 78A

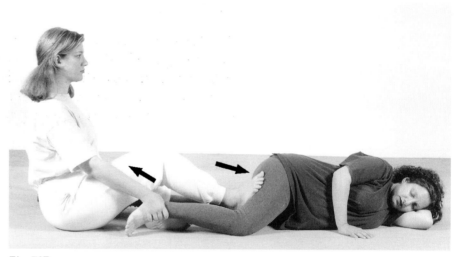

Fig. 78B

78. Sit between the client's legs and hold the ankle of the bent leg in your hand. Press the sole of your foot into the posterior thigh of the client's bent leg, starting just superior to the knee, pressing half way up the posterior thigh and then back to the knee in positions 1, 2, 3, 2, 1. With each press of the foot, simultaneously pull at the ankle creating a force/counter-force and a deepening of the compression.

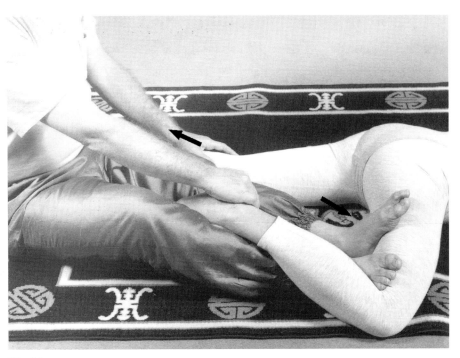

Fig. 79

79. Place the foot of the client's bent leg under the knee of your outside leg and hold at the ankle. With your other foot, press from half-way up the posterior thigh to the attachments of the hamstring muscle and back down to mid-thigh in positions 1, 2, 3, 2, 1. With each foot press, lean back, pulling at the ankle.

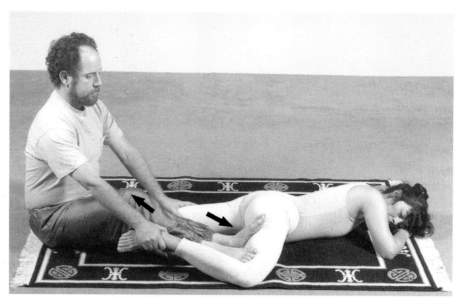

Fig. 80

80. Move the client's foot from beneath your knee, still holding at the ankle. Alternate feet while pressing with both feet into the client's posterior thigh. Simultaneously, lean back and pull at the ankle with each press of the foot.

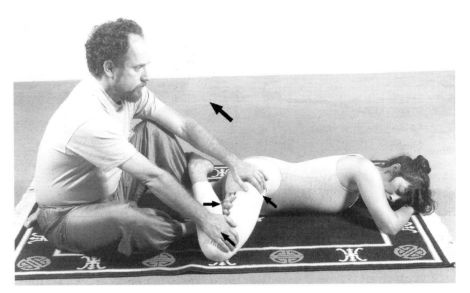

Fig. 81A

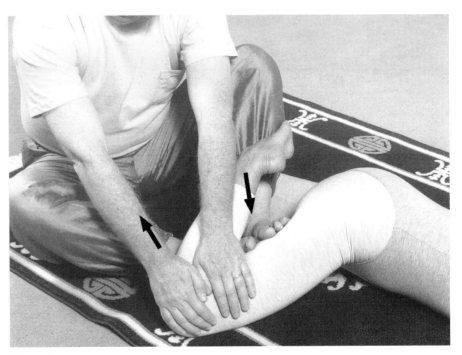

Fig. 81B

81. Place your feet side by side on the posterior mid-thigh of the client. The client's lower leg rests against your shin bone. Reach across the client's thigh and press into the Sen lines of the upper thigh with your fingertips.

Hook your fingers across the thigh, lean back and pull.

Make a loose fist and percuss the thigh.

Hips and back

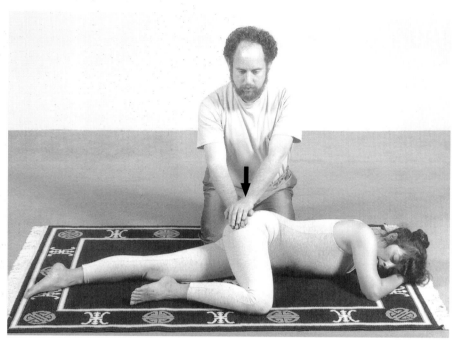

Fig. 82A

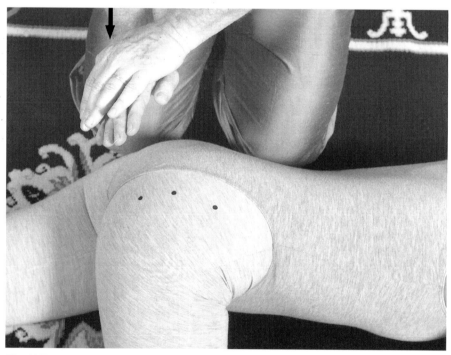

Fig. 82B

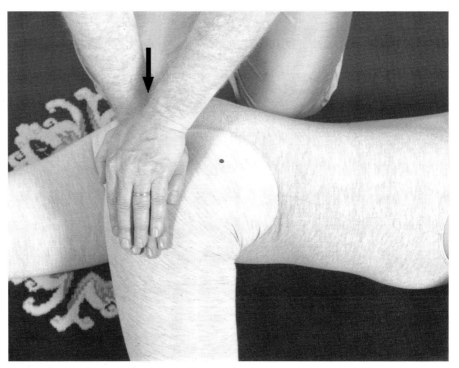

Fig. 82C

82. Kneel behind the client. Palm press the entire hip region with both hands.

Identify three points on the hip region. These points represent the endpoints of the three Sen lines on the lateral leg. The points are located in hollows of the muscles in the hip region, lateral to the sacrum, near the greater trochanter of the femur.

At each point, use the heels of your hands to make slow and deep compressions. Finish with general palm presses in the hip region for integration of the deep point work.

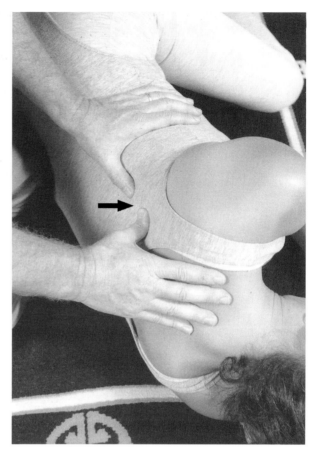

Fig. 83

83. Sit behind the client and palm press the back region that is superior to the spine, working from the hips up to the shoulders and then back down to the hips.

Thumb press on three lines on the back, utilizing the thumb-chasing-thumb technique. The first line is located along the medial border of the scapula. The second line is located in the sulcus of the sacrospinalis muscle, about one and a half inches lateral to the midline of the back. The third line is located just along the spine between the transverse and spinous processes of the vertebrae.

Treat these lines with the thumb-chasing-thumb technique in a pattern of up line 1, down line 1; up line 2, down line 2; up line 3, down line 3, and completing with palm pressing up and back down to the hips. An alternative pattern is to go up line 1, down line 2, up line 3, and palm press back down to the hips.

Continue with the thumb-chasing-thumb technique from just superior to the side of the spine at the waistline, working laterally to the mid-axillary line at the superior aspect of the iliac crest and then back to the midline of the back.

Place the client's hand and forearm behind the back. This creates an opening of the scapular region. Place one hand on the shoulder and place the thumb of your other hand on the muscle attachments on the medial border of the scapula. Pull back at the shoulder while simultaneously pressing in with the thumb of the other hand, creating a deep compression into the muscle attachments along the scapula.

Repeat this procedure all along the medial border of the scapula. Palm press around the scapula and continue along the back for integration.

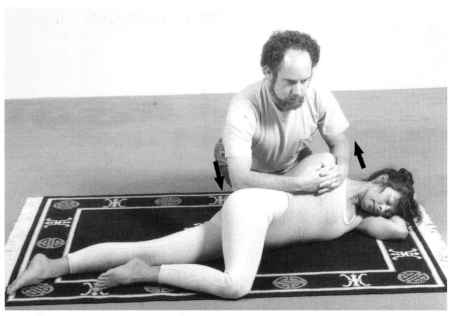

Fig. 84A

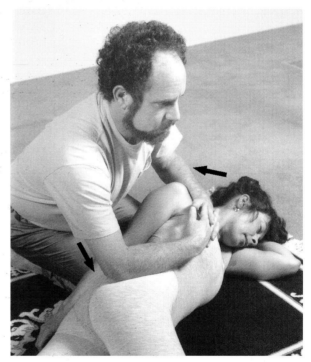

Fig. 84B

84. Interlock your fingers in front of the client's shoulder joint. Place one forearm on the client's hip. Press forward with your forearm into the client's hip while simultaneously pulling back at the shoulder joint with your other forearm, creating a lumbar stretch.

Repeat this procedure in three locations between the hip and the lower border of the rib cage, and then back down to the hip.

Arms, hands and fingers

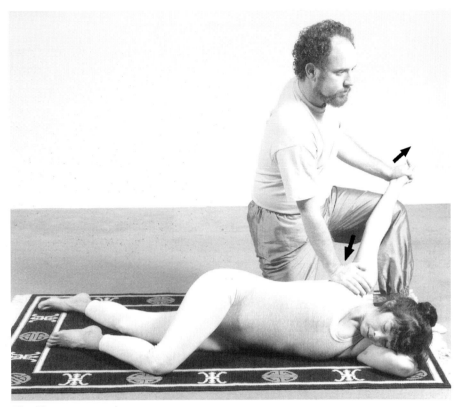

Fig. 85

85. Interlock your fingers with the client's fingers. Extend the client's arm forward above his or her head. Place your other hand at the client's axilla. Pull and extend the client's arm while simultaneously palm pressing at the axilla.

Repeat these procedures with palm presses down the side of the client's chest to the lower border of the ribcage and then back up to the axilla area, in a pattern 1, 2, 3, 2, 1.

Kneel with one leg up at a 90° angle. Place the client's arm across your bent leg, positioning the arm at a 90° angle to the client's own body. With fingers interlocked, pull the client's arm back while simultaneously pressing in at the axilla.

Release the fingers, continuing to support the client's arm across your bent leg. Palm press the medial surface of the client's arm from the wrist to the axilla and then back to the wrist.

Starting at the wrist crease, thumb press, utilizing the thumb-chasing-thumb technique, up the midline of the lower arm to the elbow. On the upper arm, thumb press in the muscle superior to the humerus bone working up into the axilla. Thumb press back down the arm to the wrist.

Palm press up the arm to the axilla.

In the axilla, palpate the pulse of the axillary artery. Place the heel of your hand firmly into the pulse, obstructing the blood flow for up to 10 seconds. Slowly release the artery and palm press back down the arm to the wrist. *The obstruction of the pulse is contraindicated with any condition of heart disease.*

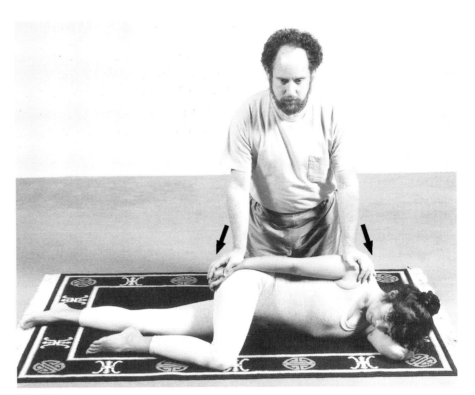

Fig. 86A

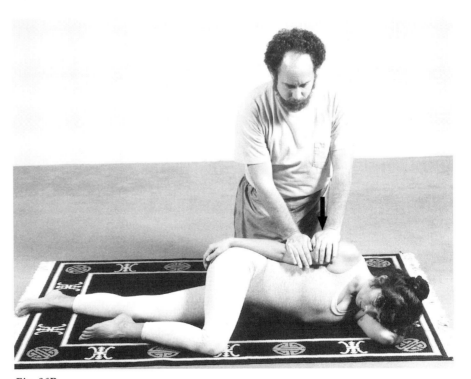

Fig. 86B

86. Place the client's arm, palmar surface down, along his or her side. Hold at the client's wrist and shoulder and stretch the arm three times.

Palm press the lateral surface of the entire arm.

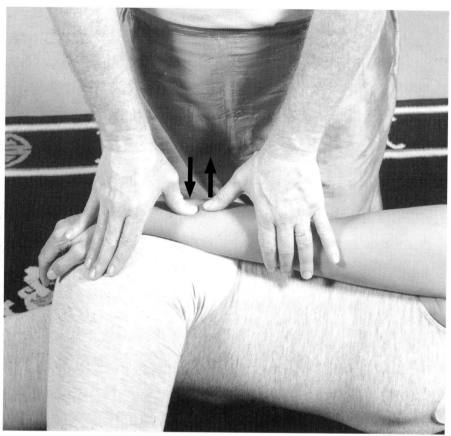

Fig. 87

87. Use the thumb-chasing-thumb technique on the center line of the lateral surface of the lower arm and posterior to the humerus bone on the upper arm, pressing up to the shoulder and then back down to the wrist. Palm press the arm for integration.

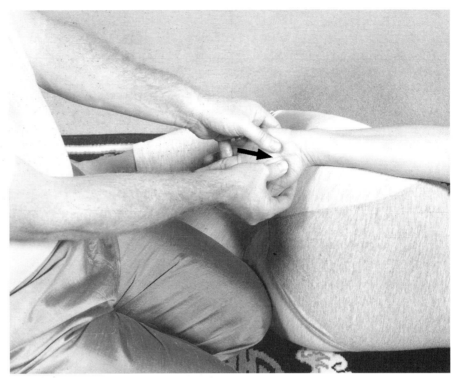

Fig. 88

88. Kneel at the client's hips, facing the head. Rotate the client's hand medially so that the palmar surface is facing up, the back of the hand resting on the hips. Using the heels of both hands, massage the palmar surface of the whole hand.

Interlocking fingers with the client, thumb press into six points on the palmar surface of the hand.

Use the heels of your hands to massage the palmar surface of the client's hand.

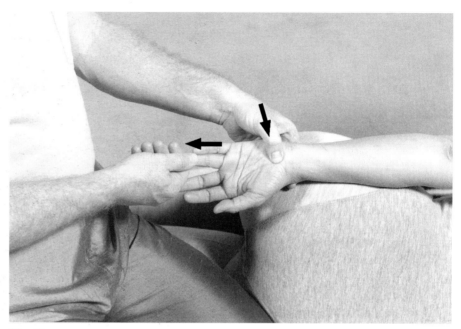

Fig. 89

89. Thumb press at the mid-point of the wrist crease. Thumb press into the palm of the hand and when the phalange bones of the thumb are reached, switch to thumb and finger circles out to the tip of the thumb. At the thumb tip, pinch and pull the thumb.

Return to the point at the middle of the wrist crease, thumb press this point and continue with the thumb presses into the palm directed toward the index finger. Where the phalange bones of the index finger begin, thumb and finger circle out the finger to the tip, completing with a pinch and a pull at the finger tip.

Repeat all of the same procedures for the other fingers.

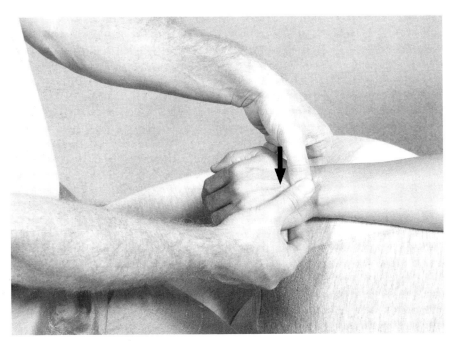

Fig. 90A

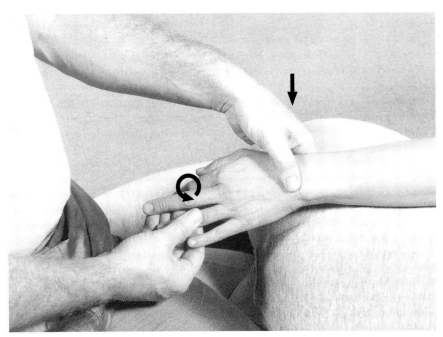

Fig. 90B

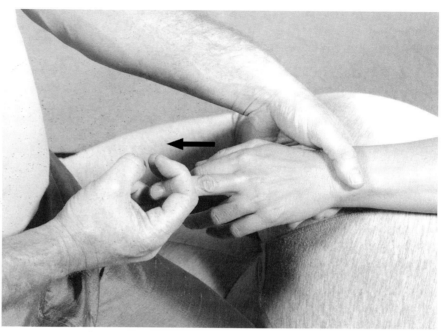

Fig. 90C

90. Rotate the client's hand, placing the palmar surface down. The client's arm rests across his or her own hip. Utilizing the heels of your hands, massage the back of the client's hand.

Thumb circle from the point on the midline at the wrist crease between the radius and ulna and the carpal bones, working distally in the grooves between the carpal bones between the thumb and index finger. At the beginning of the phalange bones of the thumb, finger and thumb circle along the thumb to the tip.

Grasp the thumb, rotate the thumb, then lean back to stretch the thumb.

Return to the point at the wrist and repeat the same procedures for each of the other fingers.

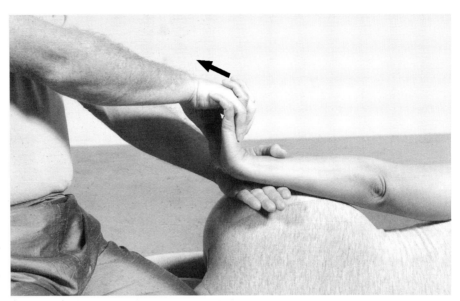

Fig. 91A

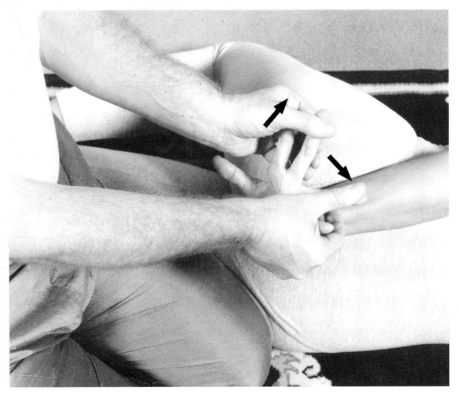

Fig. 91B

91. Hold the client's wrist with one hand and interlock the fingers with your other hand. Rotate the wrist five times clockwise and then five times counter-clockwise. Lean back three times, pulling and stretching the entire arm.

Squeeze the client's fingers with your fingers and lean back, disengaging your fingers from the client's fingers. Slowly stretch the client's fingers apart, holding two fingers at a time with each hand.

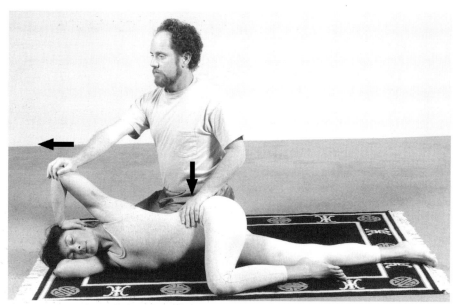

Fig. 92A

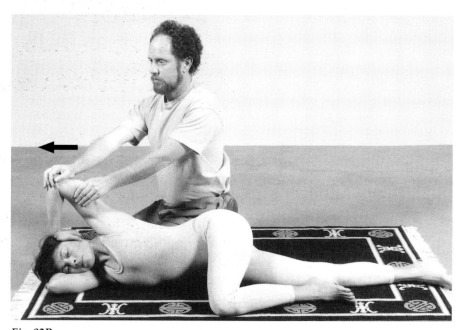

Fig. 92B

92. Raise the client's arm, placing the hand of the client over his or her own ear, with the fingers pointing back toward the shoulder.

Place one hand on the elbow and the other hand on the client's hip. Press the elbow forward toward the crown of the head while pressing on the hip, creating a stretch along the midline of the client's side. Repeat the stretch.

Keeping one hand on the elbow, massage the triceps muscle of the arm, pulling the muscle slightly away from the bone. Bring the arm back along the client's side and shake the arm for relaxation.

Stretching techniques

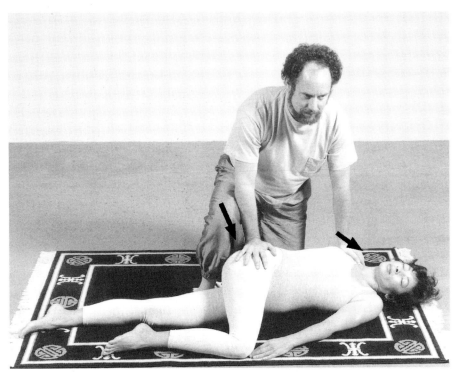

Fig. 93

93. Kneel at the client's back. Place one hand on the upper shoulder and one hand on the gluteal muscle of the bent leg. Simultaneously, press the shoulder towards the floor and the hip of the bent leg forward in the opposite direction, creating a lumbar stretch and twist.

Press at positions from the gluteus down along the iliotibial tract of the lateral thigh while simultaneously pressing at the shoulder. This is done very slowly and deeply. Most of the stretch is accomplished by pressing the shoulder toward the floor.

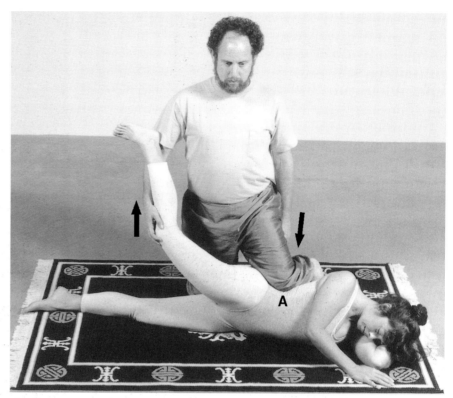

Fig. 94A

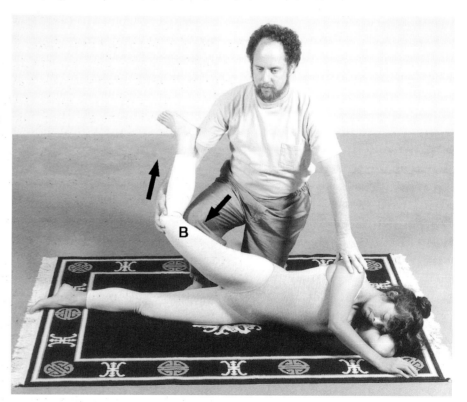

Fig. 94B

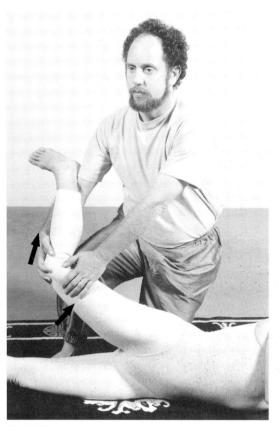

Fig. 94C

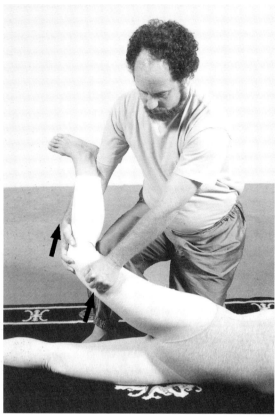

Fig. 94D

94. Kneel at the back of the client. Take the top leg in your arm with the hand holding at the knee, cradling the top leg so that the foot and upper leg will be resting against the upper arm. Place the other hand on the client's shoulder. Your knee (A) is placed in the lower back, but is not pressing inward. The procedure is accomplished by pulling the bent leg back and slightly up. This pull will create a stretch and simultaneously bring the knee deeper into the area of the back.

Place knee (A) in three positions from the lower rib area to the top of the iliac crest. Press three positions, 1, 2, 3, and then back into positions 2, 1. If the back area is small, only two positions will be done.

Then remove knee (A) from the back and place knee (B) into the posterior thigh of the bent leg of the client. With knee (B) placed on the thigh, pull the leg back. This results in a deep compression being made into the back of the client's thigh.

Work from just superior to the knee up to the gluteus in three positions, in a pattern 1, 2, 3, 2, 1.

Continue holding the client's leg in your arm and with the other hand reach around and hook the fingers into the Sen line of the upper leg of the client. Pull and lean back, working the Sen line.

After working the line, create a loose fist and percuss the thigh of the bent leg of the client. Then release the client's leg and place it on the floor.

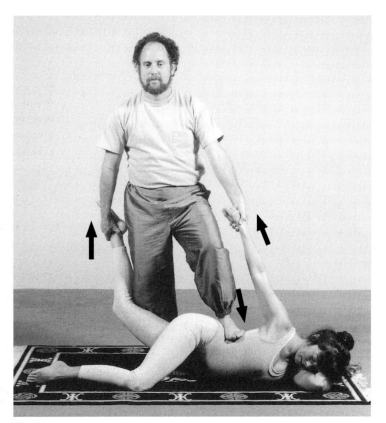

Fig. 95

95. Stand up holding the ankle of the lower leg and the wrist of the superior arm. Place your foot at the waist region of the client. Hold the arm stationary as you lift the leg. As the leg is lifted, make a slight downward pressure with the foot into the back. It is the lifting of the leg that primarily creates the deepening of the compression with the foot into the back.

Work from the waistline up toward the lower border of the twelfth rib into positions 1, 2, 1.

Set the leg down, lift the other leg and repeat the pulling of the leg and the pressing with the foot while continuing to hold the same arm.

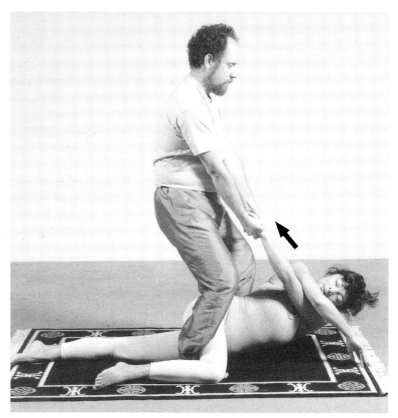

Fig. 96A

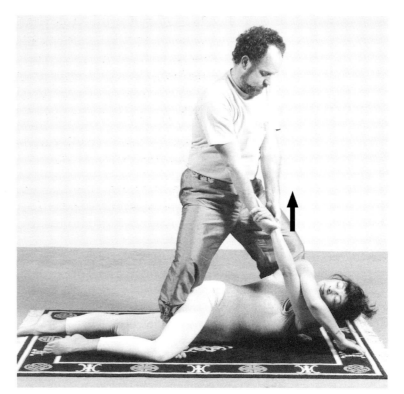

Fig. 96B

96. Remain standing, facing the client's head. Step forward so that one foot is between the client's legs and the other is outside of the legs.

Reach down, hold at the wrist, lean back and pull. This lifts the client's body slightly off the futon. The lifting is repeated three times.

Repeat all procedures from 64 through 96 with the client on their other side.

97–99. Repeat procedures 47– 49 on pages 85–87.

5 Client in prone position

Feet and legs

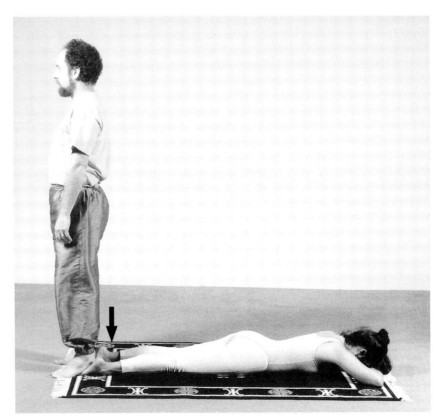

Fig. 100

100. The client lies in a prone position. Stand at the client's feet with your back to the client. Use the soles and the heels of your feet to work into the bottom of the feet of the client.

Alternating feet, work deeply and firmly and then more softly.

Turn, facing the client's head; now, using the balls of your feet, work soft, harder, and again softly, into the bottom of the client's feet.

Repeat this many times.

Kneel down and put your knees into the feet of the client and your hands at the ankles for support. Shifting your weight from side to side, work your knees deeply into the bottom of the feet. Finish with palm presses on the bottom of the feet for integration and relaxation.

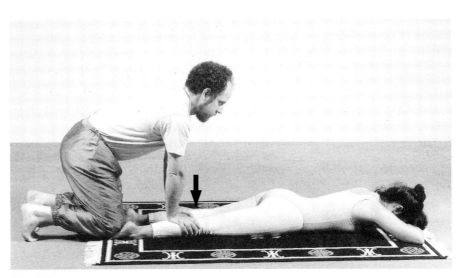

Fig. 101

101. Do walking palm presses up and down the back of the legs from the feet to the ischial tuberosities. Repeat.

Thumb press from the Achilles tendon up the mid-line of the calf, across the popliteal fossa of the knee, and along the back of the hamstrings to the ischial tuberosity. Hold a deep thumb press at the ischial tuberosity where the hamstrings attach. Thumb press back down the legs.

Palm press up and down along the entire back of the legs for integration.

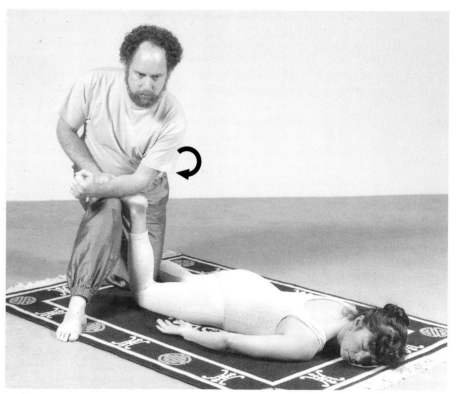

Fig. 102A

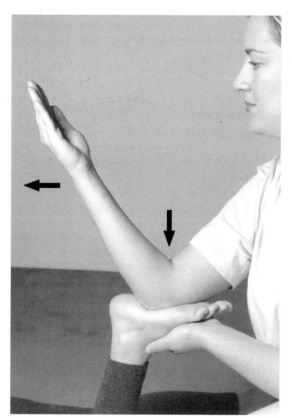

Fig. 102B

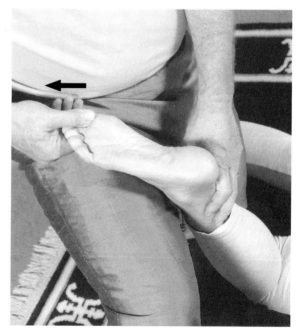

Fig. 102C

102. Kneel on one leg at the feet of the client. Raise the client's leg and place the top of the foot across your thigh. Roll the forearm over the entire foot with the thigh creating a counter-force.

Deep elbow press into the six points on the bottom of the foot. The release is achieved by bringing the forearm forward, not by lifting the elbow off the foot. Integrate by rolling the bottom of the foot with the forearm. Gently pound with a loose fist on the bottom of the foot.

Thumb presses on five lines on the bottom of the foot, beginning just anterior to the heel in the arch at point 3 (described in procedure 4 on page 38. Thumb press through the soft part of the foot, switching to thumb circles at the metatarsals, circling out each digit one at a time. For the little toe, do finger circles along the lateral aspect of the foot. Integrate the presses and circling by rolling the bottom of the foot with the forearm.

Point the foot upward and do thumb presses on the dorsal aspect of the foot, starting at the acupoint Stomach 41 Jiexi, then work down the channels between the tendons with thumb presses. Upon reaching the phalanges of each digit, do thumb and finger circles out to the end of each digit and then press at the tip.

Palm press on the top of each foot for integration and then thumb press along the medial aspect of the foot just below the bones.

Hold the ankle with one hand and do rotations of the foot, five times clockwise, five times counter-clockwise. Grasp the foot on the medial aspect, twisting and leaning back, working positions 1, 2, 3, 2, 1. Continue with pulling, massaging and opening the joints of each individual toe and popping the toes if they are able.

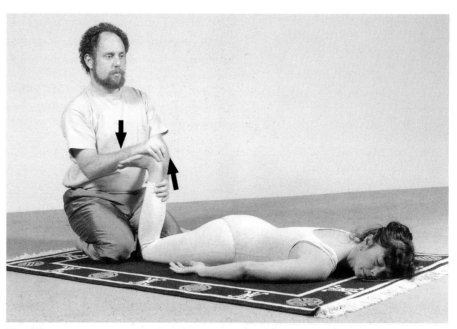

Fig. 103

103. Hold the heel in the palm, toes against the forearm, then bring the forearm downward, lifting at the heel, giving a deep stretch to the Achilles tendon.

Upon completion of these procedures, go back to the beginning of 102 and repeat all the procedures on the other foot.

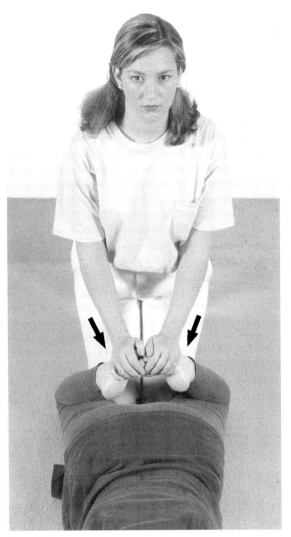

Fig. 104A

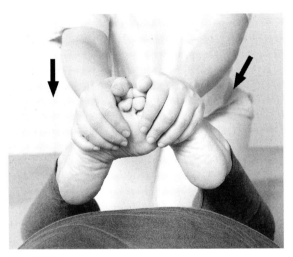

Fig. 104B

104. Place your hands at the client's ankles, pressing the feet toward the gluteus. Repeat this three times.

Shifting your hands, move upwards toward the toes and roll the toes over while pressing the feet forward toward the gluteal region. The first press is soft, the second is with medium pressure and the third is firm.

Open the space between the knees slightly, cross the feet, pressing the feet toward the gluteus three times in the pattern soft, harder, and soft.

Reverse the feet so the upper one is now on the bottom, and lean forward pressing. Position yourself on your knees, shifting your weight forward, keeping your arms straight.

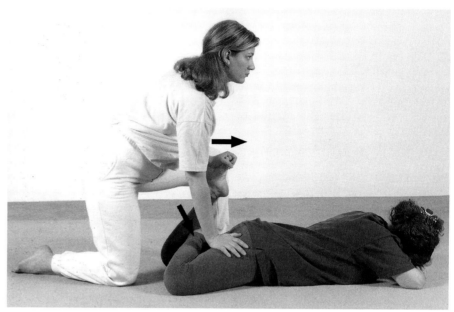

Fig. 105

105. Place one of the client's feet behind the knee on his or her other leg and then push the raised foot toward the buttock region. Simultaneously with each push forward, palm press the hamstring area of the bent leg, working in positions 1, 2, 3, 2, 1.

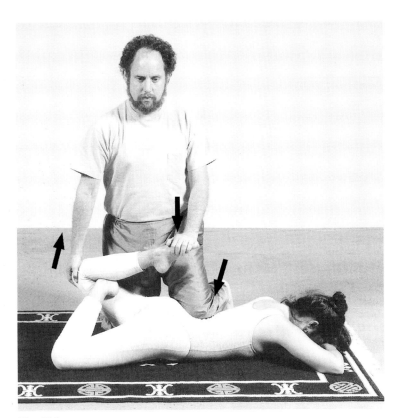

Fig. 106

106. Continue holding the raised foot in one hand and move to a position alongside the client. Place your knee gently onto the region of the client's waist. Place your other hand around the knee of the raised leg and lift the knee, bringing the foot closer to the buttocks. This lifting creates a downward vector of the knee on the client's back. With each lift of the client's knee, shift your knee from the waist up toward the lower ribs and then back down to the waist, working positions 1, 2, 3, 2, 1.

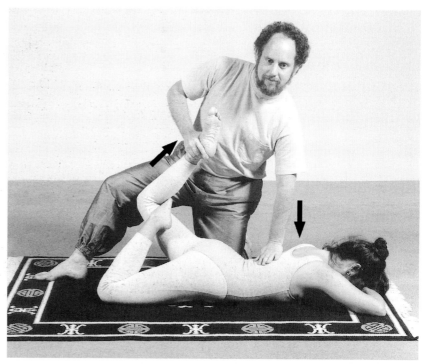

Fig. 107

107. Move your knee off the client's back and place your hand in the lower back region. Holding at the ankle with the other hand, lift the foot up. This lift of the foot and leg creates a downward force with the hand in the lower back. Three positions are pressed with the hand in the lower back from the sacrum to the lower border of the ribs.

At the completion of 107, change legs and go back to 105.

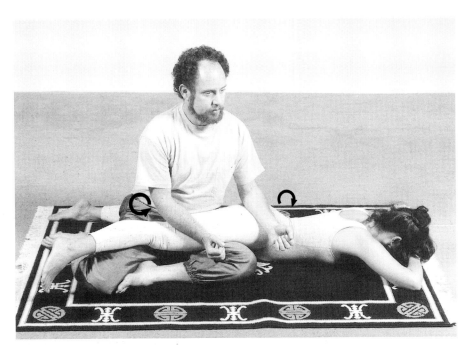

Fig. 108A

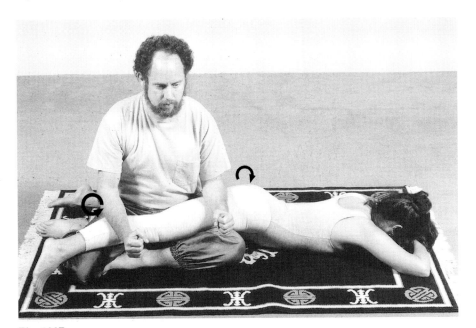

Fig. 108B

108. Sit between the client's legs with your own legs bent. Your forward forearm rests at the client's waist and the other hand is holding at the ankle. Pulling at the ankle and rolling the forearm on the back, a stretch is created.

Release at the ankle and bring this forearm onto the thigh and place the other forearm on the low back. Simultaneously, roll with both forearms in opposite directions, creating elongation.

Next, use one forearm to work on the upper thigh and one on the lower leg, rolling in opposite directions creating a compression and a stretch.

Bring the hands together to do a chopping percussion along the back of the thigh and the leg, working distally, then proximally and again distally.

Turn to the other leg, staying seated between the legs of the client and repeat the procedures on the other leg.

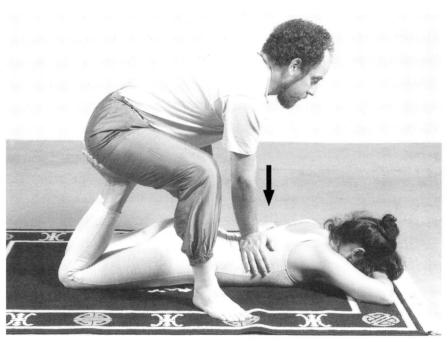

Fig. 109A

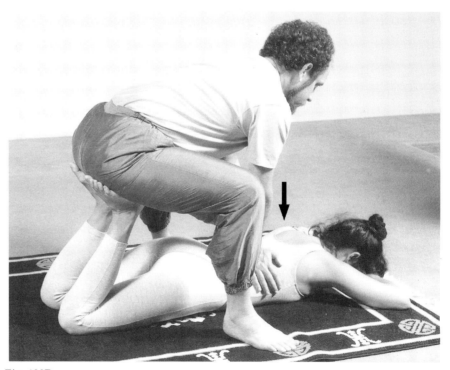

Fig. 109B

109. The client remains in a prone position. Bend the client's lower legs upwards at 90°, feet parallel to the floor. Sit on the soles of the client's feet. Place your feet in the vicinity of the client's waist. With the palms of the hands adjacent to the spinous processes of the vertebrae, palm press from the waist up along the spine to the level of the third thoracic vertebra and then palm press back down to the sacral region. Repeat the palm presses a number of times.

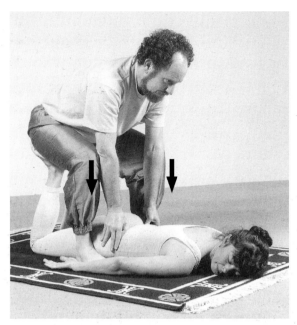

Fig. 110A

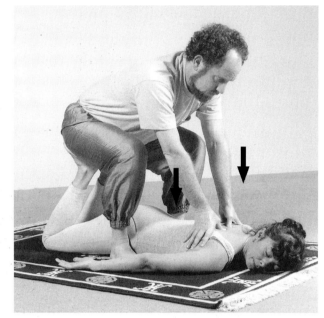

Fig. 110B

110. Remain seated on the client's feet and thumb press from the midline out along the waistline and then back to the midline. Continue with thumb presses lateral to the spine up to the level of the third thoracic vertebra and then thumb press back down toward the waist. Upon completion of the thumb presses, integrate the detailed thumb work with palm presses up and down the entire back.

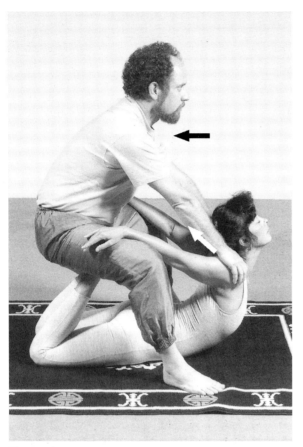

Fig. 111A

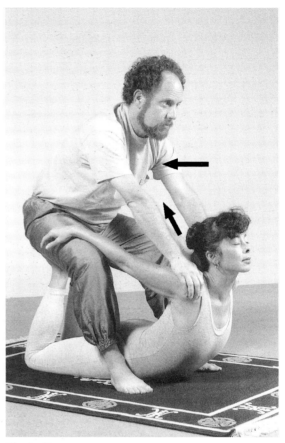

Fig. 111B

111. Remain seated on the client's feet, now placing the client's hands across your thighs. Lean forward and wrap your hands over the client's shoulders. Shift your weight onto your heels and, keeping your arms straight, pull the client up into a bow stretch. Repeat this stretch three times.

Back and shoulders

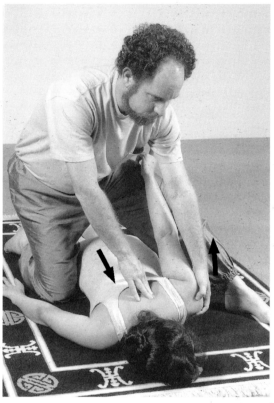

Fig. 112A

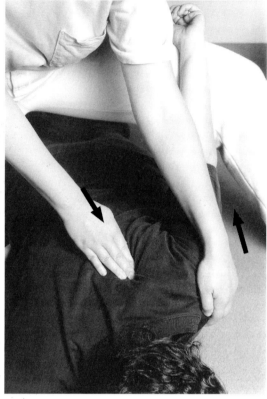

Fig. 112B

112. Come off the client's feet and kneel straddling the prone client, placing the client's left arm across your raised left knee. Reach around with the left hand, lift the left shoulder while palm pressing with the right hand the area around the scapula. Place the right fingers along the medial border of the scapula along the attachments of the muscles. Simultaneously lift the shoulder up and press in with the thumb giving a deep compression along the muscle attachments of the scapula.

Work the thumb presses from the medial superior angle of the scapula down to the lower border of the scapula at the level of the seventh thoracic vertebra, pressing in with the thumb while pulling the shoulder back and up.

Palm press the entire scapular area for integration and then finish with gentle palm or finger circles all around the vicinity of the scapula.

Set the raised arm down and repeat all the procedures on the other arm.

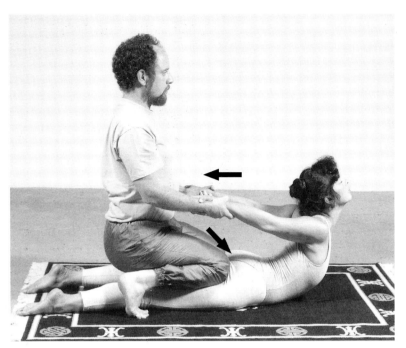

Fig. 113

113. Kneel on the back of the client's legs, placing your knees at the attachments of the hamstring muscles (at the acupoint Urinary Bladder 36 Chengfu). Leaning forward, palm press up the back, across the shoulders and down the arms to the hands, which are placed at the client's side.

Pick up the client's hands. Grasp one another's wrists. With knees still placed firmly into the hamstring attachments, lean back and pull the client's torso up off the futon. After approximately 10 seconds, lower the client's upper body. Re-position your knees slightly lower on the thighs, lean back and pull at the wrists, lifting the torso off the futon. Lower the client's body, shift the knee position again to about halfway down the thigh, and lean back pulling at the wrists. Repeat the pulls, going proximally in positions 2 and 1.

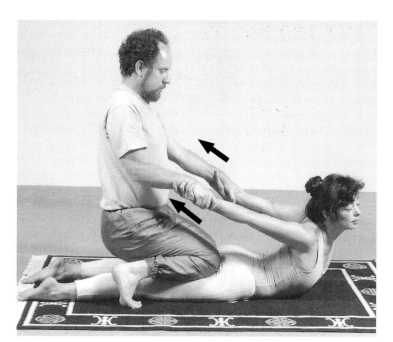

Fig. 114A

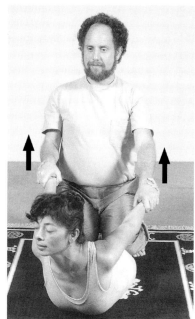

Fig. 114B

114. Repeat the three pullbacks with the knees in three positions. With each pull, while the torso is raised, gently swing the client's upper body from side to side by pulling back on one arm at a time.

Lower the client's body, release at the wrists and remove the knees from the thighs. Palm press with the hands up the arms, across the shoulders, down the back and continue down the legs to the feet, integrating the entire back of the client's body.

Stretching techniques

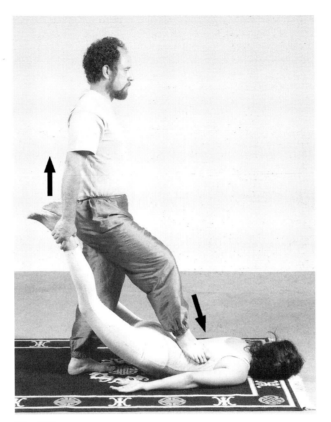

Fig. 115

115. Stand up and hold the ankles of both legs. Gently place one foot on the low back of the client just above the sacrum. The foot is arched over the spine, delivering a slight pressure with the heel and the toes. Lift the legs up, creating a stretch, and allow a small amount of pressure to be delivered through the foot into the low back.

Lower the legs slightly, change the foot position proximally. The foot positions are from just above the sacrum to the lower border of the ribs. At each new foot position, lift the legs. Depending on the size of the client, there will be three or four foot positions.

This procedure is contraindicated for client's with low back pain, disc problems or who have had previous back surgery.

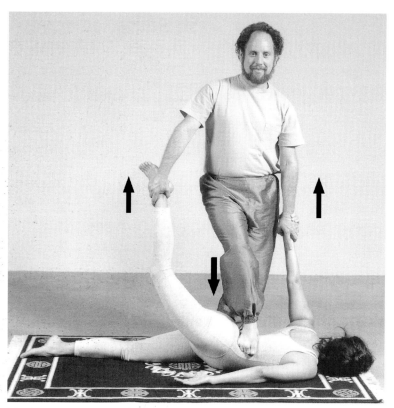

Fig. 116A

116. Lower the legs, move to the client's left side, reach down to hold the right ankle and lift the right leg with your right hand. The client's left arm is raised and held at the wrist. Place your right foot on the low back. Pull the leg slightly up; this increases the pressure delivered downward by the foot. With each lift of the leg, change the foot position in the lumbar region.

This procedure is contraindicated for client's with low back pain, disc problems or who have had previous back surgery.

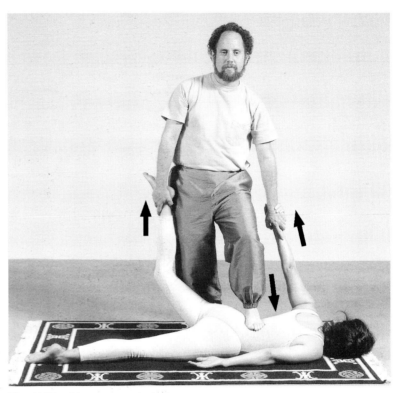

Fig. 116B

Let the right leg down and lift the left leg while continuing to hold the left arm. Repeat the leg lifts while the foot shifts positions on the low back.

This procedure is contraindicated for client's with low back pain, disc problems or who have had previous back surgery.

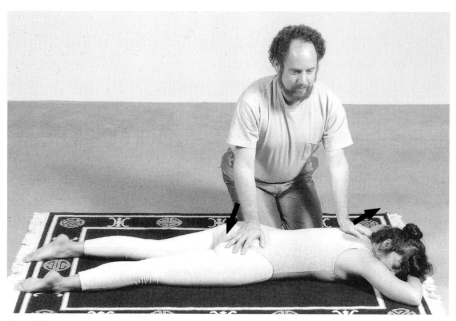

Fig. 117

117. Kneel by the client's side. Place the left hand over the left scapula and the right hand across the sacroiliac joint on the client's right side. Simultaneously, press down and away with both hands, creating a diagonal stretch and elongation of the back. Repeat the stretch three times.

Release the hands, move to the other side of the client, place the hands as before but now with the right hand over the right scapula. Repeat the stretch three times.

Continue with gentle palm and finger circles around the spine and the entire area of the back. Finish with palm presses over the entire back region.

118. The client rolls over into the supine position. Palm press the feet and up and down the legs a number of times. Stand, lifting the client's legs, and place the legs along your abdomen. Holding at the wrists, pull and lean back, bringing the client's torso up and forward. Repeat the procedure three times. (See Figs. 47, 48, 49.)

119. The practitioner and client have an interlocking grip at the wrists. The client crosses his or her legs into a half lotus position, with the legs resting against your lower legs. Lean back and pull the client up and forward. Lower the client and repeat the pull. The third time, pull the client up and take a few small steps backward, bringing the client into a seated position.

6 Client in seated position

Shoulders, neck and back

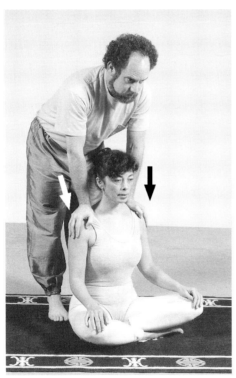

Fig. 120A

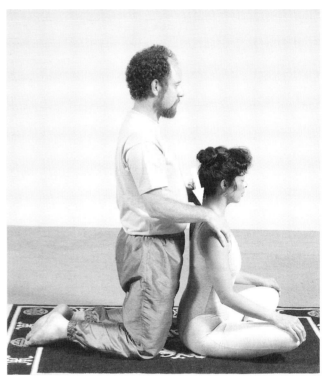

Fig. 120B

120. The client is in a seated position, legs crossed. Kneel or stand behind the client with your legs resting against the client's back to give support. Lean forward with straight arms, palm pressing the upper trapezius region. Palm press from the nape of the neck laterally to the acromial extremity at positions 1, 2, 3 and then back at positions 2 and 1.

Thumb press the same area of the upper trapezius, working on both shoulders simultaneously. Palm press for integration.

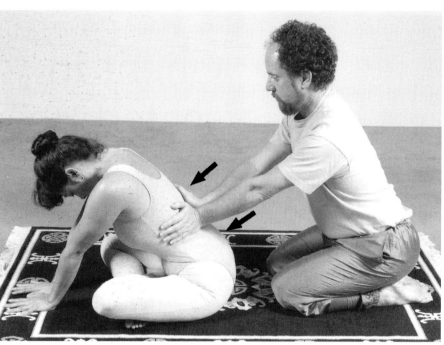

Fig. 121

121. The client's hands are placed palmar surface down on the futon in front of him or her, to create a counter-force. Palm press the entire back, down and up.

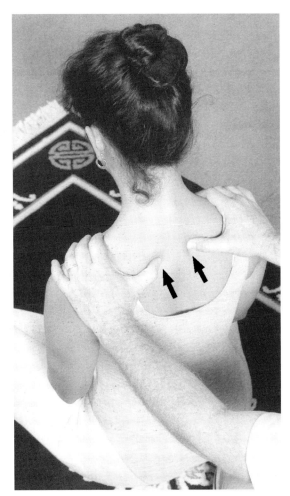

Fig. 122

122. Thumb press down the back on either side of the spine. Just superior to the sacrum, thumb press laterally and then medially around the waist at the belt-line. Thumb press up the back to the nape of the neck. Complete with palm presses down and back up the entire back for general relaxation and integration.

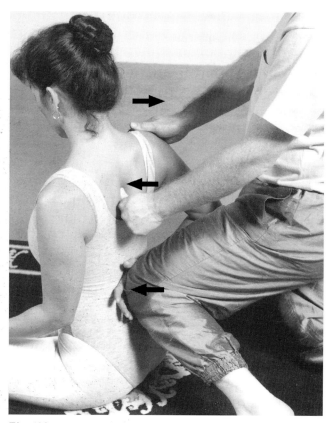

Fig. 123

123. Bring the client's right hand to rest in the area of the low back. Hold the hand in place by your left knee pressing into the palm. Your right hand is placed on the front of the shoulder joint. Palm press the entire region of the right scapula.

Press your thumb or fingers along the medial border of the scapula while simultaneously pulling the shoulder back to deepen the compression. Work the entire scapular region in this manner.

Use finger circles and palm presses to relax the whole area. Complete this section by kneading and squeezing the triceps muscle of the upper arm.

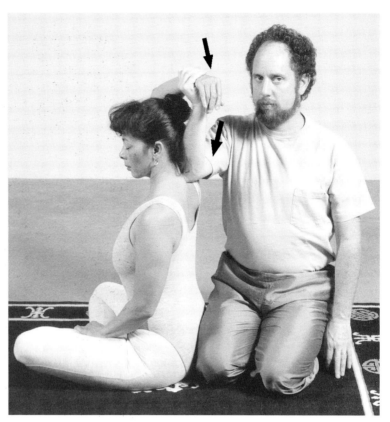

Fig. 124A

124. Sit at a 90° angle to the client's back, with your right side supporting the client's back. Lift the client's right arm at the wrist with your right hand. Place your right elbow on the attachments of the levator scapulae at the superior medial border of the scapula. Slowly pull the client's wrist toward the opposite shoulder. This pull creates a downward vector with the elbow into the muscle attachments.

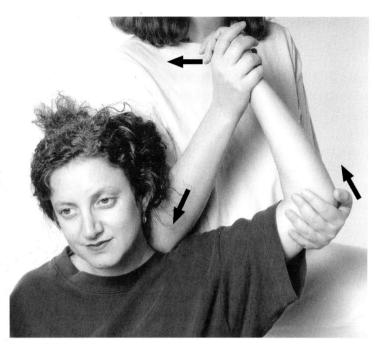

Fig. 124B

Release the pull at the wrist, re-position your elbow closer to the spine, and again pull at the wrist.

Repeat the procedure with the elbow positioned along the medial border of the scapula and on the upper trapezius muscle.

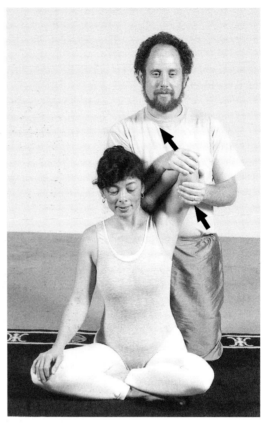

Fig. 125

125. Place the client's hand on the back of his or her own neck. Take your arm and lay it over the client's forearm so that your hand grasps over the elbow. Pull back and slightly up on the elbow and with the other hand use the fingertips to work the triceps muscle of the upper arm. Knead the muscle and compress the muscle into the bone. Finally, make a loose fist and percuss the triceps muscle.

Upon completion of 125, return to 123 and repeat all the procedures on the other arm.

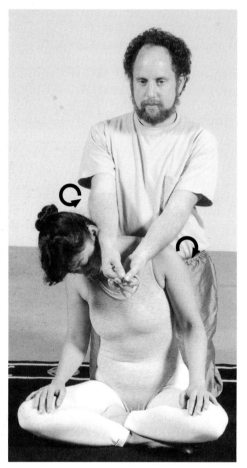

Fig. 126

126. Place your right forearm against the left side of the client's head, just below the ear. Your left forearm rests on the client's acromial extremity. Interlock your fingers. Rotate the radius bones of your arms, creating an extension and moving the client's head laterally, creating a stretch of the neck. Repeat the stretch three times.

Release and repeat the procedure on the other side. Gently rub the neck and shoulders for relaxation.

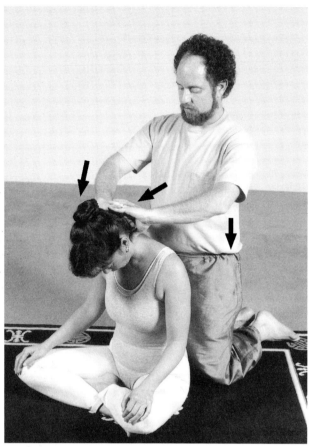

Fig. 127A

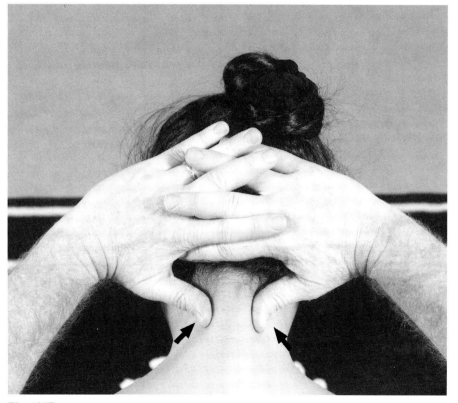

Fig. 127B

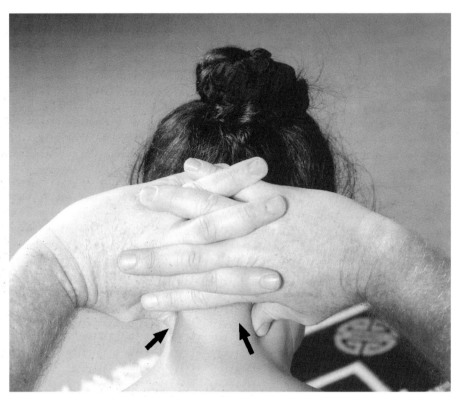

Fig. 127C

127. Interlock your fingers, rotate your palms so that the thumbs are pointing down. Place the thumbs against the trapezius muscles on both sides of the neck. Slowly drop your elbows, thus creating a vice-like effect with your thumbs squeezing into the muscles of the client's neck. Start with the thumbs just below the occipital ridge and work down to the region lateral to the seventh cervical vertebra. Work down the neck, then back up and then down, being careful not to exhibit excessive force.

Keeping the fingers interlaced, place the heels of the hands against the side of the neck and squeeze, creating a deep kneading sensation. Work along the entire neck region. Finish with finger circles on the neck for relaxation and integration of the deep neck work.

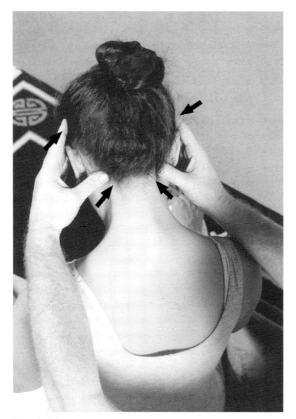

Fig. 128A

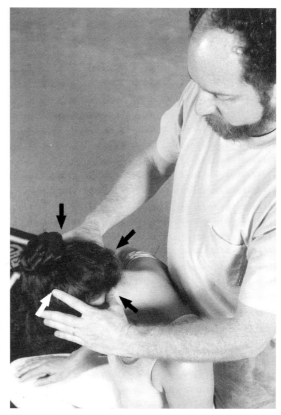

Fig. 128B

128. Hold the client's forehead with one hand and thumb press with the other hand along the occipital ridge from the midline to the mastoid process.

Switch hands and thumb press the other side. An alternative approach is to work with both thumbs simultaneously, supporting the head with the fingers placed on the scalp.

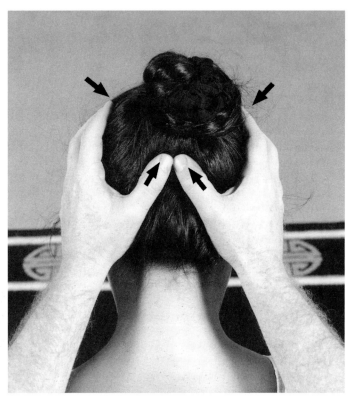

Fig. 129

129. Begin thumb presses in the hollow just below the occipital protuberance and continue up along the midline of the head to the crown. Thumb press back down into the hollow and then back up to the crown.

Stand up and continue with the thumb presses from the crown to the hairline and back to the crown of the head. The thumb press technique can be either thumb-on-thumb or thumb-chasing-thumb.

Make gentle finger circles through the entire scalp, 'shampooing' the entire scalp area, and complete by scratching the scalp.

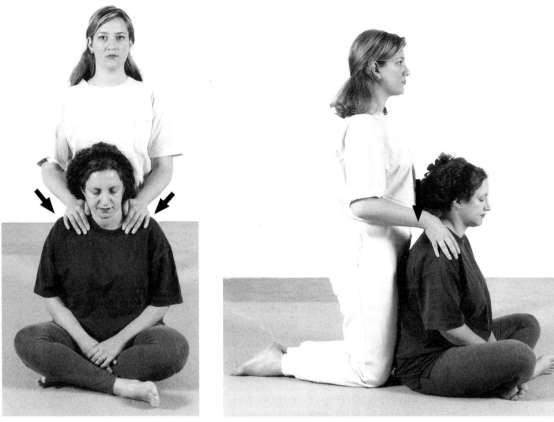

Fig. 130A   *Fig. 130B*

130. Palm press the shoulders, continue with thumb presses on the shoulders, and then repeat the palm presses. Finger circle the muscles of the neck.

Face

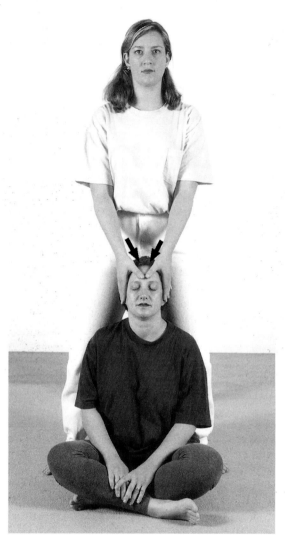

Fig. 131

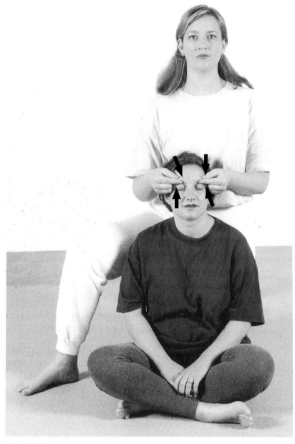

Fig. 132A

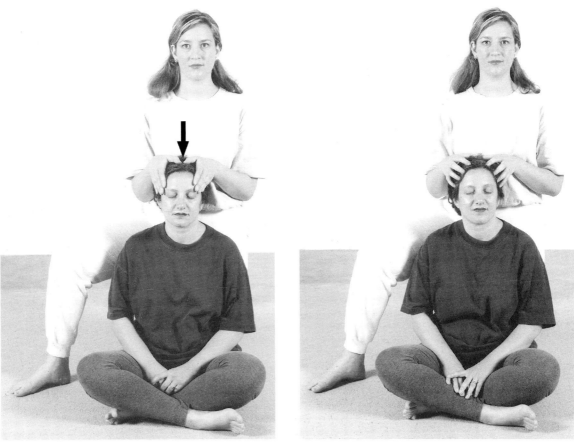

Fig. 132B

Fig. 132C

131–132. (The work on the face can be done using thumb presses and/or finger circles). Treat across the forehead, along the eyebrows, around the orbits of the eyes and into the masseter muscles of the jaw. At the completion of each line, palm circles in the region of the temples are utilized for integration and relaxation.

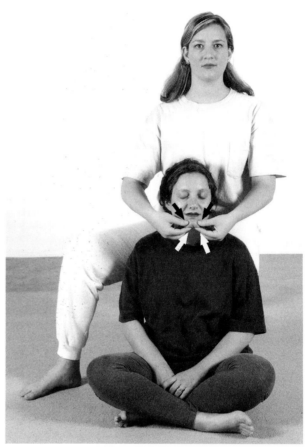

Fig. 133

133. Use the thumbs and index fingers to massage the chin.

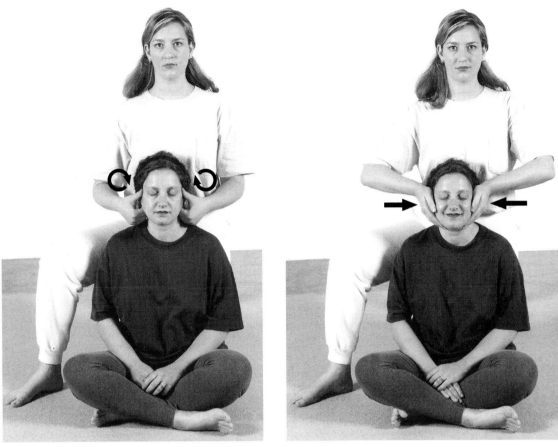

Fig. 134A   *Fig. 134B*

134. Work around the ears with thumb presses and finger circles. Use the thumbs and index fingers to firmly massage the auricle of the ear.

Cup the hands and cover the ears, obstructing the hearing for up to 30 seconds. Release gradually and repeat twice more. Finish with gentle finger circles around the ears, the sides of the head and the temples. Palm circle in the templar region.

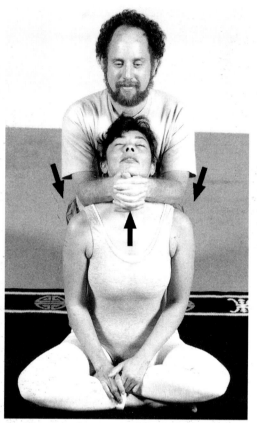

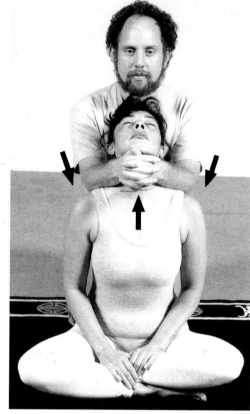

Fig. 135A *Fig. 135B*

135. Kneel behind the client, extend your arms across the shoulders and interlock your fingers under the client's chin, being careful not to press into the client's throat. Press down with your forearms into the shoulders and lift at the chin with the interlocked fingers, creating an extension, lifting the head slightly back. Repeat three times.

Repeat the same chin lifting technique and now rotate the head first to the left side then to the right side, moving very slowly. The last lift is with the head facing straight ahead. Finish this section with gentle finger circles on the shoulders and neck for relaxation.

Stretching techniques

136. The client clasps his or her hands together, interlocking the fingers behind the neck. Stand behind the client placing your hands around the elbows and gently lift up and back to open and expand the area of the shoulders and chest. Press your thigh in the client's back as you pull the elbows back, enhancing the stretch.

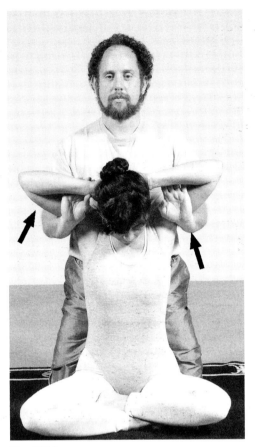

Fig. 137A

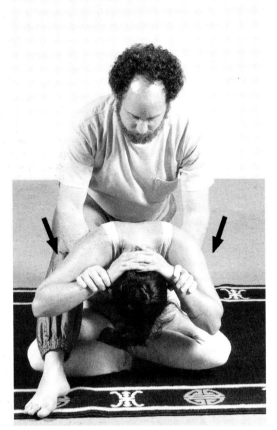

Fig. 137B

137. The client continues with interlocked fingers positioned at the back of the head. Kneel down and bring your hands underneath the client's upper arm, through the space between the upper arm and the forearm, and hold at the wrists. Bring the client's body forward and back three times.

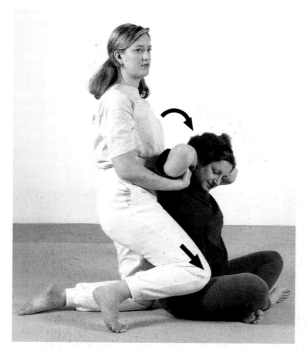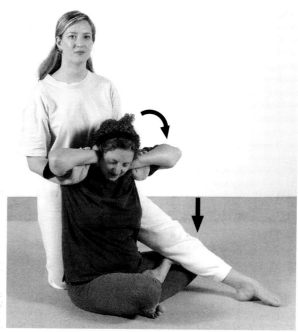

Fig. 138A   *Fig. 138B*

138. The same interlocking position with the arms and hands is maintained. Shift to the side and fix the client's thigh with your knee. Bring the client's torso forward and then rotate and bring the client's torso back up to the side opposite where the leg is held in place. This creates a twist and stretch.

Lower the torso forward, shift the position of the knee proximally on the thigh and repeat the twist and lift.

Reposition the knee on the thigh a third time and repeat the procedure.

Change sides and repeat the three stretches on the second side.

An alternative approach is to hold the client's leg in place with your outstretched leg.

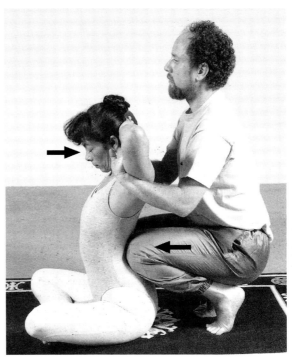

Fig. 139

139. Continue holding the arms in the same position. Take up a squatting position, up on the toes. Place your knees on the client's back, just below the scapula. Pull the client slowly back creating a compression with your knees.

Bring the client slightly forward, shift the knee position down and pull back.

Change the position of the knees a third time, locating them now just above the sacrum, and pull the client back into the knees.

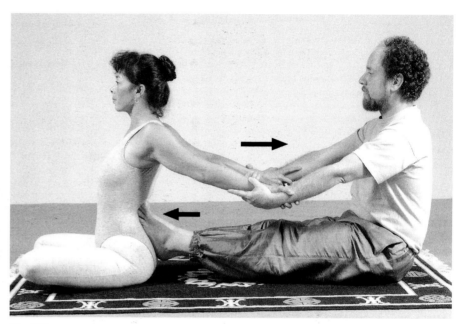

Fig. 140

140. Sit down. The client's arms extend back and practitioner and client hold each other at the wrists. Place your feet into the low back of the client and push forward with your feet while simultaneously pulling back with the arms, creating a force/counter-force. There are three positions on the back where the feet are placed, starting at the low back/sacral region and continuing up to the area just below the scapula.

Repeat the pushes with the feet in positions 1, 2, 3, 2, 1 while simultaneously pulling the arms.

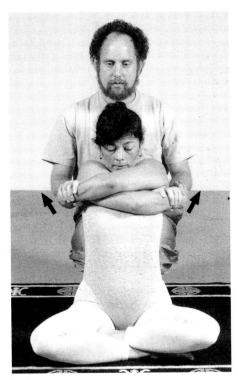

Fig. 141A

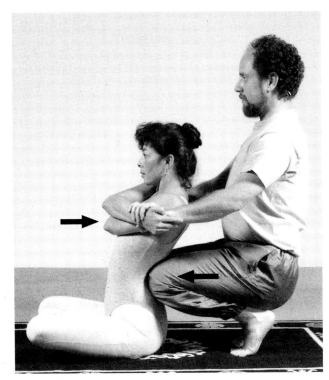

Fig. 141B

141. The client gives himself or herself a big hug by wrapping the arms around the body. Squat behind the client, placing your knees on the client's back, just below the scapulae. Hold the client at the wrists. Pull the client back creating a force that presses the knees into the back.

Repeat with the knees in three positions from the lower border of the scapula down to the waistline, repeating the procedures in positions 1, 2, 3, 2, 1.

Ending the session

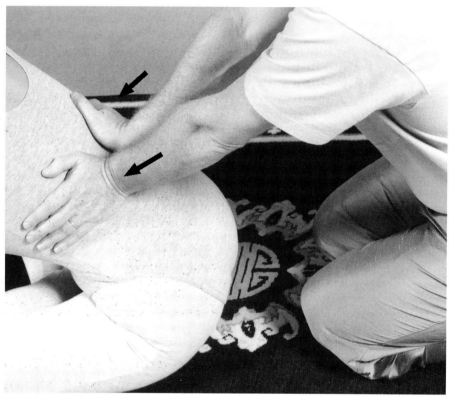

Fig. 142A

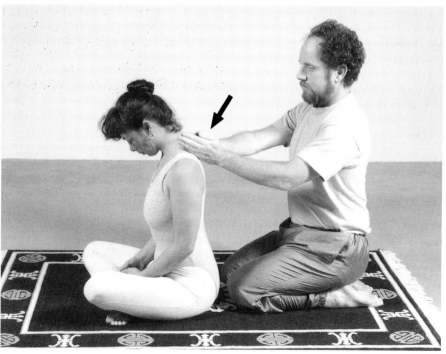

Fig. 142B

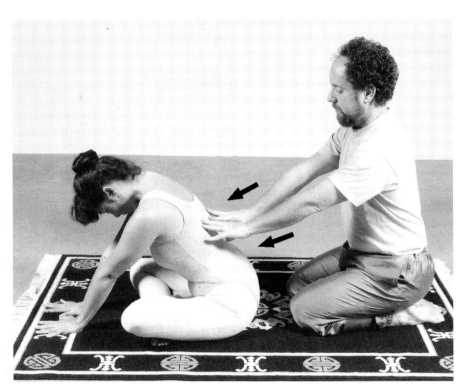

Fig. 142C

142. Kneel behind the client. The client leans forward and braces with his or her hands in front, on the futon. Palm press down the back with hands together. Continue with alternating palm presses on the whole back.

Put your hands together, pressing the fingertips and the heels of your hands together. Continue with chopping percussion with the hands down and up the entire back, being careful not to exert undue pressure over the kidneys. Finish with gentle brushing movements with the fingertips across the entire back for calming and integration.

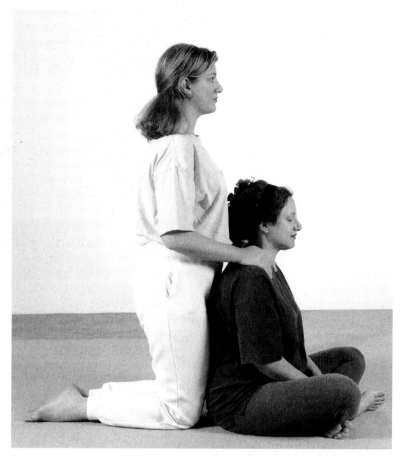

Fig. 143

143. Gently place your hands on the client's shoulders. Share a final moment of quiet and stillness. OM NAMO. With gratitude, the session is completed.

Conclusion

7 Conclusion

'Through study, practice and experience, we come to know and embody this work.'

Thai massage can be utilized as a healing modality for a particular complaint or can be used to provide a deeply relaxing and rejuvenating body therapy experience. A session of Thai massage can take a short amount of time or can last for hours. If a practitioner were to attempt to use every procedure taught in this book, a session would take approximately 4 hours to complete. This is impractical in the Western cultural context. The practical, clinical application of this work involves choices being made by the practitioner based on the client's needs and desires. Certain procedures will be included or left out of a session depending on the goals and intentions of a session. The practitioner should never hurry any aspect of this work in order to include something in a specific amount of time. The work is always done slowly, evenly, and continuously.

This book presents comprehensive instruction in Chiang Mai (northern style) of traditional Thai medical massage. There is also a southern style that varies somewhat from the northern and is taught at Wat Po and practiced in southern Thailand and especially on the islands in the south. Further academic research and study in the entire field of Thai medicine is called for. The application of these massage techniques for specific complaints is the subject of further writing. Also, a detailed study of Thai herbal medicine, food cures, and spiritual practices as related to healing warrants research and publication. I hope to be able to accomplish some of this work in the future and I also hope that this book might encourage others in academia and in the realm of natural medicine to further study of the traditional medicine of Thailand.

Om Namo Shivago . . . 'I venerate the compassionate Father Doctor with good conduct'.

References

1. Brun V, Schumacher T 1987 Traditional herbal medicine in northern Thailand. University of California Press, Berkeley
2. Boriharnwanaket 1995 Metta. Triple Gem Press, London
3. Smith M 1957 A physician at the court of Siam. Oxford University Press, Oxford
4. Maciocia G 1989 The foundations of Chinese medicine. Churchill Livingstone, Edinburgh
5. Kaptchuk T 1983 The web that has no weaver. Congdon & Weed, New York

Further Reading

Bechert H, Gombrich R (eds) 1984 The world of Buddhism. Thames and Hudson, London

Chopra D 1991 Perfect health. Harmony Books, New York

Golomb L 1985 An anthropology of curing in multiethnic Thailand. University of Illinois Press, Chicago

Heyn B 1992 Ayurvedic medicine. Harper Collins, New Delhi

Mulholland J 1977 Thai traditional medicine: a preliminary investigation. Australian National University Press, Canberra

Riley JN, Mitchell JR, Bensky D 1981 Thai manipulative medicine as represented in the Wat Pho epigraphies. Medical Anthropology 5(2)

Setthakorn C 1989 Nuad Bo'Rarn workbook. Foundation of Shivago Komparaj, Chiang Mai

Xinnong C (ed) 1996 Chinese acupuncture and moxibustion. Foreign Language Press, Beijing

Appendix

Mantra

A twice daily aspect of the training program in traditional Thai massage at the Old Medicine Hospital in Chiang Mai is a ceremony known as 'Wai Khru'. Every morning prior to the beginning of instruction and every afternoon at the completion of class, there is a period of chanting and prayer. A long prayer is chanted by the Thai instructors and Thai students, followed by a shorter prayer that is chanted by everyone, including the foreign students. Below is the prayer, known as a mantra, that everyone chants. A mantra is a mystical formula of invocation or incantation. The literal meaning of the mantra is less important than the general spirit it seeks to invoke. The sounds themselves constitute what are considered to be sacred syllables that call forth blessings, charms, and spells. The mantra was never fully explained nor translated by the instructors. It was described as a tribute to the 'Father Doctor' and as a means for the students to focus themselves for the study and practice of the work.

I had the desire to delve into the mantra more thoroughly, and therefore sought out a resource to assist in this pursuit. Fortunately, I had a resource from my undergraduate days at Oberlin College. In fact, we had become acquainted in college during the month long meditation retreat where I had first been exposed to Thai Therevada Buddhist meditation. Geoffrey DeGraff had gone to Thailand after graduating from college in 1971. Over the years, he remained in Thailand, learned the Thai and Pali languages, and eventually took vows and became ordained as a Buddhist monk. In the first part of the 1990s, Geoffrey, now known as Than, was sent to America to become the Abbott at the Metta Forest Monastery near San Diego, California. I have included here Geoffrey's brief commentary and literal translation of the mantra.

Note: In paragraph 2, the word *nagas* appears, Nagas are earth spirits that are serpent shaped and consume evil energy and evil spirits.

A mantra to Father Doctor Jivaka

1. Om namo Jivako silassa aham karuniko sabba-sattanam osatha-dipamantam papaso suriya-candam Komarapacco pakasesi vandami pandito sumedhaso aroga-sumano homi (3 times)

2. Piyo deva-manussanam   Piyo brahmanamuttamo
   Piyo Naga-supannanam   Pinindriyam namami'ham

3. Namo buddhaya na-won na-wien na-sathit na-sathien ehi-mama na-wien na-we na-pai tang-wien na-wien mahaku ehi-mama piyong-mama namo buddhaya

4. Na-a na-va roga-byadhi vinasanti (3 times)

Commentary and translation

This mantra, like all mantras, is virtually impossible to translate, as it is composed of an ungrammatical mixture of Pali and Thai words and half-words. The following is a transliterated version following the standard transliteration schemes for Pali and Thai, plus what can be pieced together from the individual words and phrases. The grammar is unchanged – there is a general feeling in south and south-east Asia that the less grammatical and intelligible the mantra, the more effective it is.

1. Om = aum, namo = homage, silassa = to a virtuous person, aham = I, karuniko sabba-sattanam = compassionate for all living beings, osatha-dipamantam = medicine with candles, papaso = to or of evil, suriya-candam = the sun and moon, Komarapacco = Jivaka's surname, pakasesi = he announces, vandami = I pay respect, pandito = a wise man, sumedhaso = to or of an intelligent man, aroga-sumano homu = May I be free from disease and happy.

2. This verse is from a magic poem about the virtues of the Buddha. The translation reads: He is dear to devas and human beings, most dear to Brahmas, dear to nagas and garudas. I pay homage to the one whose sense faculties are fresh and clear. (The form of the poem requires that all the lines in this stanza begin with the syllable *pi*.)

3. Namo buddhaya = homage to the Buddha, na-won na-wien = *na* here is taken from *namo, won-wien* is Thai for 'spinning around', sathit-sathien = is Thai for 'firmly established', ehi-mama = come to me. The rest of this passage consists of half-words combined with words explained above.

4. roga byadhi vinasanti = diseases and illnesses are destroyed. If the verb were *vinasantu*, the sentence would read 'May diseases and illnesses be destroyed'.